Bariatric Recovery

Discover the Power of The Bariatric Gastric Sleeve Weight Loss Surgery Recovery Diet - Get Back to Perfect Health and Wellness with Kent McCabe Emma Aqiyl

Dr. Jonathan Brown
Dr Patt Wright
Sarah Levine M.D.
Patt Vince Harrison
Redford E. Gordon

Table of Contents

PART 1

Introduction

This book has a very wide range of people it can help. Whether you're just considering Bariatric surgery, trying to figure out if you'd be a good candidate, or if you have the date set for surgery and you want to know what to expect and how to prepare, want to know about post-op care and recovery, or how to maintain your body after surgery, this can help anyone from the beginning steps all the way until months after. You'll find out what the requirements are for surgery and if you can qualify, the different kinds of procedures and the pros and cons of each one, how you'll need to prepare and what diet restrictions you'll have after surgery. This book will also include foods that you can and can't eat before and after surgery along with a meal guide for after your procedure. This will be the beginning of a whole new lifestyle for you so congrats on taking the first step to making that change!

Chapter 1: What? Who? And Why?

What is Bariatric surgery? By definition, Bariatric surgery is a surgical procedure performed on the stomach or intestines to induce weight loss. Weight loss is achieved by wrapping a gastric band around the stomach to reduce its size or by re-routing the small intestine to a small stomach pouch. The procedure causes weight loss by restricting the amount of food the stomach can hold. The most common types of procedures are Gastric Bypass, Gastric Sleeve, Adjustable Gastric Band, and Biliopancreatic Diversion with Duodenal Switch (BPD/DS).

- Gastric Bypass
  - This is done by dividing the top part of the stomach, then dividing the first portion of the small intestine and attaching it to the top piece of the divided stomach.
  - Pros: On average you'll lose 60%-80% of your excess weight, restricts the amount of food you can consume, can lead to increased energy, positive changes in gut hormones that enhance satiety and reduce appetite.
  - Cons: It's a more complex operation compared to the other procedures, which could result to more complications, it could lead to long-term vitamin/mineral deficiencies (particularly in Vitamin B12, iron, calcium, and folate), typically a longer hospital stay is required compared to other procedures, requires following your doctor's dietary recommendations, and could lead to life-long vitamin/mineral supplementation.
- Gastric Sleeve

- o This procedure is done by removing 80% of the stomach. The new stomach holds much less than the normal stomach so there's much less calories being consumed.
- o Pros: It restricts the amount of food that your stomach can hold, induces significant weight loss in a short amount of time, and it does not require any foreign objects or rerouting the food stream, normally a short hospital stay (about 2 days), and causes changes in gut hormones that suppress hunger, reduce appetite and improve satiety.
- o Cons: The procedure is non-reversible, there is a possibility of having long-term vitamin/mineral deficiencies, and there is a higher chance of an early complication rate.
- Adjustable Gastric Band
  - o This involves putting an inflatable band around the upper portion of the stomach. This creates a smaller stomach pouch above the band.
  - o Pros: Reduces the amount of food that can go into the stomach, typical weight loss of about 40%-50% of your excess weight, it does not involve any cutting or rerouting, requires a much shorter hospital stay compared to other procedures (usually around 24 hours or you can even be released the same day), this procedure is reversible, has the lowest rate of early post-op complications, and has the lowest risk for vitamin and mineral deficiencies.
  - o Cons: This procedure has the highest rate of re-operation, it requires sticking to a strict post-op diet and going to your post-

op follow up visits, dilation in the esophagus can result if you overeat, you may experience mechanical problems with the band, procedure requires a foreign device to remain inside of your body, a higher percentage of patients fail to lose up to 50% of excess body weight, less early weight loss, and slower weight loss compared to other procedures.

- Biliopancreatic Diversion with Duodenal Switch (BPD/DS)
  - o There are two parts to this procedure. First, a portion of the stomach is removed, leaving a tube shaped stomach. Then, a large portion of the small intestine is bypassed.
  - o Pros: Average weight loss is about 60%-70% of your excess weight at a 5 year follow up which is much greater than other procedures, it is the most effective procedure against diabetes, causes changes in gut hormones that improves satiety and reduces appetite, reduces fat absorption by 70% or more, and it also allows patients to eventually eat more "normal" meals.
  - o Cons: There is a higher risk compared to similar procedures, requires a longer hospital stay, requires a very strict compliance with follow up visits and dietary/vitamin supplementation recommendations, and guidelines are critical to avoiding serious complications such as protein and vitamin deficiencies.

If you have been considering Bariatric surgery, I hope the list above has given you some things to consider when you think about which procedure would be right for you. Depending on which procedure you have done that can affect how long you're in the hospital, your recovery time and how much weight you lose after the surgery.

Who would be a good candidate for Bariatric surgery? If you are considering surgery, then there are a few things you need to ask yourself first. One of the first questions you need to ask yourself is what is your BMI? If you have a BMI over 40, then most organizations would say that weight loss surgery is a reasonable option for you, but you must be healthy enough to sustain surgery. To give you an example, if your height is 5'5" then your BMI would be 40 if you weighed 240 ½ pounds. The next question you should ask yourself is do you have any weight related medical conditions? In some cases, certain medical conditions may help qualify you for surgery, but others might make you not able to withstand the procedure. If you have a BMI of 35 or over, you may qualify for surgery if you have at least one obesity related medical condition such as Type 2 Diabetes, hypertension, gastrointestinal disorders, heart disease, non-alcoholic fatty liver disease, osteoarthritis, lipid abnormalities, sleep apnea and other respiratory disorders.

Why should you consider Bariatric surgery? Most people that are considering having these procedures done or already have had them done have tried other weight loss options and have not been successful with them. If it's at all possible to avoid surgery, then you should go with that option since all procedures are not without their own risks. Some examples of a non-surgical option to losing weight would be diet and exercise, a support group or a partner who will motivate you, supplements or weight loss medication. If you haven't tried any of these options, then you may not qualify for surgery.

We now know what Bariatric surgery is and the different procedures that are available. You should pick the procedure that will best fit your needs and consider all the risks that comes along with each procedure, along with the benefits. Some procedures have higher risks than others and some can make you lose a higher amount of weight in a shorter amount of time. You should consider both the risks and benefits when choosing one. Once you've weighed your options and you have figured out if you would be a good candidate and why you want the surgery, that will better help you in finding out which one would be the best option for you. Once you know which procedure you will be doing, we can move on to how you can prepare for you big day.

Chapter 2: Preparing for Surgery

This surgery is a big step into your new lifestyle. In order to prepare you'll have to make a few changes. First, if you are a smoker then it will be required that you stop smoking before your surgery. This will reduce the risk of some complications after surgery. If you don't quit smoking before surgery it can cause breathing problems before and after the procedure, and you'll have a higher risk of developing pneumonia. Smoking also slows down your blood flow, which means you won't heal as fast. On top of that making your recovery time much longer, that also means you are at risk of infection for a much larger period of time than you normally would have been. It's recommended that you quit smoking at least a week in advance. But even quitting just one day in advance can decrease your chances of complications, although the earlier the better. You will also need to stick to any medications your physician has prescribed you along with any dietary restrictions that were given to you. Unless given a diet to follow by your doctor, here is a diet that you should follow at least 3 weeks before your surgery.

- You should be eating at least 60 grams a day of protein.
- Eliminate all refined sugars and reduce carb intake.
- Eat healthy fats, avoid bad kinds of fat.
    - Healthy fats: Avocado, fish, nuts, olives, etc.
    - Bad fats: Butter, vegetable oil, fast food, cake, etc.
- Avoid high calorie foods.
- 48-72 hours before surgery you should be on an all liquid diet. Do not consume any solid food.

- The night before your surgery you should stop consuming all liquids and food. This allows the surgeon to operate without any interference.

You also may need to stop taking certain medication before surgery. Inform your doctor of any medication you are taking so they can tell you what is and isn't safe to be taking before surgery. Medications you may need to stop taking include arthritis medication, NSAIDS (nonsteroidal anti-inflammatory drugs such as Tylenol, Aspirin, Ibuprofen, Naproxen), and any anticoagulants (Enoxaparin, Clopidogrel, Dipyridamole, Ticlopidine, and Warfarin). Any medication that acts as a blood thinner should be removed from your diet to remove the risk of complications during surgery.

Other planning may be needed depending on the length of the hospital stay and your recovery time. These can vary based on which procedure you are having done. You may want a family member, close friend or spouse to stay with you at the hospital or at home with you for support once you are released. It is also a good idea to make home and/or work arrangements since you will be recovering for a few weeks.

You will also need to mentally prepare yourself for surgery and for life after. You need to find the root cause of your weight gain. Is it because of a health issue? Stress? Is it because of depression or a food addiction? Many people who are obese whose cause is not related to a health issue may have problems with food addiction. It is imperative that you know food addictions not dealt with after surgery can have dire consequences. You can severely harm yourself if you continue the food addiction after you have the surgery. The reason this is so important is because when you eat large amounts of food it can cause your stomach to rupture. This can happen with a normal stomach so your chances of having your newly, much smaller stomach rupture rapidly increase. Having this procedure done will not make food addictions go away. That is a lifestyle change that only you can make. You must want to change, surgery or no surgery. If you don't, you will have severe consequences to deal with.

Preparing for your procedure may be a little tough but it's preparing you for your new lifestyle ahead. Since you'll be recovering for a little while after surgery remember to take care of any responsibilities you may have over the next few weeks and to not have anything to eat or drink for the 24 hours leading up to the surgery. It may be hard to do but keep your goals in mind and let them motivate you.

Chapter 3: Your Surgery Day!

After all the time you've spent preparing, it's finally here. It's time to get your surgery! The morning of your procedure there are still a few last preparations. Any medications you are still taking should only be taken with a sip of water, anything that could be lost or is going to be taken off should be left at home, and wear something comfy. You're going to be here for a while, so you should make yourself comfortable. You've been eating a pretty restrictive diet lately and have consumed nothing at all the past 24 hours. On top of that you're probably feeling nervous. Don't freak out, it's completely normal to feel this way but knowing what to expect can help you to relax. When you arrive at the hospital, you'll sign some paperwork and get checked in, then you'll be taken back to an examination room. Here you'll do your pre-op physical, EKG (a process that records electrical activity of the heart) and have some blood/lab work done. Then a physician will come out to go over your procedure and this is when any questions you may have can be asked and answered. You'll be given an I.V. and then you'll wait until someone comes to get you. When they come to get you to bring you back for surgery you will be taken back to the operating room on a stretcher. Your family/friends that are there with you will go wait in the waiting room until you are done with your procedure. Before your surgery starts your anesthesiologist will give you a medication and you'll go to sleep.

A nurse will notify your family when your surgery is complete and the surgeon that performed on you will speak to them in the waiting room Depending on the type of procedure you had done, you'll either wake up on a stretcher or a hospital bed. You will always have an R.N. available to you and if you need any pain medication then there will be a button for you to push. Discomfort after surgery is normal but report if you feel any sudden/severe pain or shortness of breath. Some common complaints are shoulder pain, soreness on the left-side abdominal area, nausea, constipation/diarrhea, gas pain, weakness, and fatigue. Keep in mind this is just a guideline. This is a researched example to give you an idea of what to expect on the day of your surgery.

Congratulations, you made it! I'm sure you're excited and will want to know how much weight you can expect to start losing. You should ask your doctor, but your results can be varied depending on multiple factors. This depends on which procedure you had done, how much you weigh now, and how you take care of yourself from here on out will all contribute to your weight loss results. Most people lose about 60% of their excess weight after gastric bypass surgery. Now that you're done with your surgery and are now recovering, you can learn about post-op care.

Chapter 4: Post-op Care

Before we talk about post-op care, I'm going to include some side effects that you might experience after surgery and include if they are just a common side effect, or if they can seriously harm you so you'll know what to look out for.

- Constipation (common)
  - This is very common after weight loss surgery. Inform your doctor and they will instruct you on what to do.
- Gallstones (common)
  - Up to 50% of patients will develop gallstones after weight loss surgery because it develops when you lose a lot of weight in a short amount of time.
  - 15%-25% of people will need surgery to remove their gallstones after gastric bypass surgery.
  - Gallstones can also cause nausea, vomiting and abdominal pain.
- Blood clots in your lungs (serious)
  - This is rare, happening only 1% of the time but is still a possibility.
  - Although this can be life threatening, blood thinning drugs can usually prevent blood clots. Frequent activity can also prevent it.
- Bleeding in stool (serious)
  - This can appear reddish or black and is very serious. Inform your doctor immediately.

- Dumping Syndrome (common)
  - This can happen if you eat meals that are high in sugar after weight loss surgery.
- Wound infections (common)
  - This can happen up to 3 weeks after surgery.
  - Symptoms include redness and warmth, pus, and pain from the wound.
  - Requires antibiotics and could possibly need surgery.
- Leaks (serious)
  - Rare, but serious.
  - Can occur up to 5 days after surgery.
  - Symptoms include abdominal pain and feeling ill.
  - Call your doctor if you think that you are experiencing this.

Post-op care is very important, especially for weight loss surgery. As previously mentioned, you can severely harm yourself by not following certain guidelines. Dietary guidelines are extremely important to follow, and they are critical to your health, recovery and success with your weight loss journey. Vitamins and minerals are also very important to take because they will give you the nutrients that you need after your surgery. Most procedures also cause vitamin and/or mineral deficiencies so taking them will help to prevent that. It would be a good idea to incorporate some exercise into your routine, daily physical activity is important. It's recommended that you get 30 minutes each day. There are also support groups if you want some extra help to stay motivated. These groups are for people who have had weight loss surgery and would like to share advice, thoughts and concerns, ask questions, and overall give support. If you aren't comfortable with a group maybe you can find a family member or a close friend that is interested in doing this journey with you and you can motivate each other to reach your goals.

Although your surgeon will probably give you a list of recommended foods, some of the food items for a Bariatric surgery post-op diet are tea, sugar-free, non-carbonated beverages, non-acidic juices, broth (chicken, beef, vegetable) cottage cheese, oatmeal, and cream of wheat. There is a diet progression which you MUST follow. This is extremely important, if you try to eat something that is too solid too soon then you could possibly rupture your stomach. The diet progression goes clear liquids, full liquids, pureed foods, soft foods, and then finally solid foods. It could take 4-12 weeks for you to go through the entire progression. How quickly you go through it can depend on the type of surgery you had, speed of recovery, and your body's natural tolerance to the food progression. During the clear liquid diet phase, you can only drink liquids that are see through. This includes tea, water, diluted fruit juice that is non-acidic, protein fruit drinks, sugar-free gelatins, and artificially sweetened non-carbonated drinks. Once your body can handle clear liquids, you can move onto the full liquid phase. In this phase you can have protein shakes, skim milk, low-fat cream soups, low-fat yogurt, sugar-free gelatin, and sugar-free pudding. The next phase is pureed foods. This is soft food blended up to have a smoother consistency, to make it easier for your stomach to handle and does not have any chunks in it. The type of food that is included in this has a pretty large range because it doesn't have to originally be soft since it's getting blended. Next is the soft food phase and this is when you can start eating actual food again, but it needs to be easy to chew. This can include steamed vegetables, soft fruit, pasta, and oatmeal. Even though your eating soft foods it can still be hard on your stomach. Make sure your food is mushy and you've thoroughly chewed it before swallowing. It will probably take you 30-60 minutes to finish a meal if you are chewing properly. I know this may seem tedious, but it's very important that your food is completely chewed so that it is easier to digest. It may tire you now while eating but you'll thank yourself later when your stomach can digest what you've eaten. The last phase is the solid food diet. Once you can normally eat soft foods again you can move onto this phase. You should slowly add solid food to your diet and more and more will be added gradually so that your digestive system can get used to the solid food. You should still be chewing slowly and thoroughly even at this phase. Once again I know it may seem like you can handle it but your stomach is very sensitive right now and even when you move up to solid foods, especially when you move to solid foods, you'll need to chew thoroughly and slowly to take it easy on your stomach. Along with the dietary progression you should be following dietary guidelines as well so that you are getting the nutrition that your body needs. You should choose healthy foods that are low on fat and high in protein. Remember to drink plenty of fluids throughout the day but avoid drinking with meals. One of your biggest concerns is going to be making sure you're eating enough protein. Protein is not something that the body replenishes. For women, the daily requirements are 50-60 grams. For men, the requirements are 60-70 grams. You may need to take protein supplements to meet your daily requirements after surgery.

Something that you'll have to be slow and consistent with is your fitness after surgery. It's important to keep you body healthy and this will help you work towards your goal. After surgery if you are planning on exercising, take it very SLOW. There are countless people that tried to do too much, too soon after their surgery and ended up bedridden for a week or more. This will set you back quite a bit as far as your fitness goals are concerned so if you really want to keep progressing then you will be extra careful to not go too far. In the days immediately following your surgery, the medical team will be telling you to walk as much as you can. You should spend the first few days at home getting up out of bed and walking around the house. Any physical activity is good, get up and walk around if you're bored or to watch T.V. It seems like it's pointless but it's really not. Any kind of exercise will increase the blood flow in your body. By moving around, this tells your brain that your muscles are being used and this will burn calories. The only thing that you are able to consume right now is a protein shake, so you aren't consuming any substantial amount of calories. When your body burns calories and they aren't being replenished then it will have to pull those calories from somewhere and start dipping into your fat reserves, this burns fat! At a few weeks out form your surgery you can start doing easy exercise. Such as leg lifts, shoulder rolls, any sitting exercises, and you can continue walking too. You can just increase the distance. Once you're about a month down the road from your surgery, you'll be able to crank it up a notch. Some exercises you should be able to do at this point are water aerobics and cycling. After a few more months you should be able to move onto strength training. This includes yoga, squats, and lunges. You can try going to the gym or do a workout from home. Start out with something easy and work your way up. If you choose to go to the gym you can start out with a smaller pair of weights and make a workout routine. If you choose to stay at home, it can be as simple as having a yoga mat and some resistance bands.

With any post-op care, whether it's eating or exercising, please take it slow! It may seem like things are progressing way too slowly, but your body needs this time to get used to doing things again after all it's been through.

Chapter 5: Life After Surgery

The first few weeks after surgery you'll probably be a little sore and be on an all liquid diet. You'll start walking around even if it's for 5 minutes at a time. You shouldn't try to do anything more physically demanding than that. Even a few months after surgery you'll still need to take it easy. You'll be eating more solid foods at this point and able to do more physically. At 6 months after surgery you'll have had a bit of weight loss. If you had gastric bypass surgery, then you will have lost 30%-40% of your excess weight. With gastric band surgery you lose about 1-2 pounds a week, so at this point would be anywhere from 25-50 pounds lost. One year after surgery you will have lost a significant amount of weight. The most dramatic changes happen within a year of your surgery. You are likely to your goal weight. With gastric banding you will have lost 100 pounds. If you haven't lost this amount it's important that you find the cause and make sure you are doing everything you can to contribute to your weight loss.

There are some changes you'll need to make with your personal life too after surgery if you wish to be successful with your weight loss journey. You'll need to tell your friends and family that it's very important for you to eat healthy from now on and stick to your smaller portions. It's much easier to stick to a healthy lifestyle when you have the support from everyone around you. But it can be that much harder if they don't. If your spouse, friends and family are still eating unhealthy and large portions then that can be really difficult to keep up with your healthy lifestyle. It's even possible that some people in your life might be jealous of you and might try to make you feel bad when you start to lose weight and they are still overweight. You should surround yourself with a group of people that support you and make it easier for you to live your new, healthy lifestyle. Losing weight can have a lot of impact on the relationships in your life. Hopefully for the better, but not always. How your relationship with your significant other if affected can depend a lot on how the relationship was before surgery. Did you have a good relationship? Was it not so good? If it was a bad relationship, they may have made you feel bad for being obese or maybe they liked your old weight and don't want you to change. If this is the case, they may become controlling and overly jealous when they see you losing weight. If you had a good relationship, then it should only strengthen your bond. If your S.O. decides to get healthier with you then that's great! If you have children then this choice will affect them too, but for the better! If you have a younger child, then you will help them develop healthy eating patterns and get used to eating healthy foods. If you have an older child, maybe even one that is overweight themselves, then you can help them make the changes earlier on in their life that you are now.

Chapter 6: How to Maintain Your Body and Stay in Shape

You'll have to learn how to take care of your new body. Not just right after surgery, but for the rest of your life. You'll have to be consistent in eating healthy and exercising if you want to stay in shape, you're going to have a whole lifestyle change! To stay consistent with working out, you should find a workout routine that works for you. Don't try to make yourself do something that you don't like to do. If you aren't a runner, try swimming. If you don't like lifting weights, try calisthenics. Find something that you can see yourself enjoying and progressing in. Plan your workout for the next few days in advance or every Sunday/Monday plan your workouts for the week ahead. You'll need to make a workout plan that you'll stick with. Set simple and easy to reach goals the first time around. Don't try to accomplish too much or you could hurt yourself or give up too early when you don't finish what you planned to. I know you're excited about losing weight and you want to get started, but you are more likely to lose less weight by planning to do more than you can actually accomplish. It's great to have big goals and you should always strive to progress and push past your limits to reach your new goal, but when you bite off more than you can chew you can't swallow! In other words, it's very easy to get discouraged in the beginning if you set impossible goals for yourself. It may take some time to see results in the beginning and that can be really hard to deal with. You're putting in so much work and you don't get to see any results yet. Believe me, if you push past this hump you WILL see results and by then you will have developed a habit eating healthy and working out. It will be so much easier to remain consistent once you do this. You've overcome the hardest obstacle, it is now a habit for you, and you've started to see results! Seeing the results that you've worked so hard for is the best motivation that you could receive.

Keeping a healthy diet is another goal you'll want to make sure you're reaching. Planning your meals ahead of time is a great way to avoid sneaking in snacks, overeating and binging an unhealthy meal. It takes the guesswork out of cooking and it'll probably save you from splurging at the grocery store. I would suggest planning your 3 big meals everyday and then also prepare for 2 healthy snacks a day. One in between breakfast and lunch, and one in between lunch and dinner. For your meals you should come up with an entrée, and for your sides and snacks you should make an approved healthy list to pick from. This list can of course grow if you find any snacks or sides you would like to try that are healthy. It's your choice if you wish to only prepare for the meal or if you would like to meal prep. Meal prepping is helpful because you don't have to put any thought into what you eat after it's prepped for the week because they are completely planned out, cooked, and ready for you to grab when it's time to eat. But if you like to cook or just don't want to cook all of your meals the next few days or week then you can stick to only planning what you're going to eat. You'll still have to make your food, but this is still helpful by taking the guesswork out of what you're going to eat. You shouldn't have any snacks after dinner because you are probably winding down for the day which means you aren't using as much energy from your body as you would in the middle of the day. Calories put into your body that aren't used will be stored and then turned into fat. Stick to liquids after dinner that way if you feel snacky you can drink some tea or water and you won't be putting very many, if any, calories in your body but your stomach will feel fuller.

Once you get started in your new lifestyle you will eventually need to progress past what you're doing now. Set new goals the same way you did your first ones. This time you are more acquainted with what you can accomplish which will allow you to set goals that will push you, but not set a goal that is unreachable. Although you should set goals that are realistically within your reach, you should never let anything get too easy and never let yourself get bored. That can go for more than just working out. You should try new things and create new challenges for yourself. Goals don't have to only be fitness related, they can be anything that helps to improve any part of your life. Your goals could include starting a new happy or progress in your job. There are so many things that we can do with life, you should never get bored! If you don't know what to do, that itself could be your goal. To go out and discover what you like. Maybe you have a creative side you never knew about. You could start writing, drawing, painting, or try out photography. Maybe you want to meet new people and make friends, or maybe you want to travel. There is so much out in the world to do that there should never be a reason to be bored. This is a great way to have a happy and healthy lifestyle before or after surgery. Staying busy and doing things that you love with people you care about can help depression, prevent overeating and unhealthy eating since you are staying busy, all of these things will help you overcome obesity.

Surgery or not, a big step in staying healthy and fit is consistency. It's going to be very hard for your body to lose weight if you aren't keeping up with your workouts and eating healthy. Pick a meal plan and a workout routine that fits your wants and needs and works with your schedule. Since your whole day is already planned it takes out any of the guesswork. You have a whole plan laid out you just have to go out and do it. Since you were productive, you'll feel happy and accomplished at the end of the day.

PART 2

Introduction

Congratulations on downloading *Gastric Sleeve Solution: The Ultimate Bypass Surgery Weight Loss Surgery Recipes for Rapid Recovery and Healing,* and thank you for doing so. Deciding on having gastric bypass surgery is a monumental decision and it is one that should be made with care and consideration. The surgery can assist you on your way to a healthier lifestyle and a lower body weight, but you must also be willing to put in additional effort in eating a nutritious diet and exercising regularly.

The following chapters will discuss how to determine if you are a good candidate for weight loss surgery, what surgical options may be available to you, and what your recovery period will look like. There will also be a section at the end of the book devoted entirely too tasty, nutritious recipes that will help you on the road to recovery after surgery. These recipes will be based around specific foods that are known for healing the body and helping you to get the best nutrition you can as you recover. They are also recipes that were created with small portions in mind, specifically for patients who have undergone gastric bypass surgeries. Nutritional information will be included with each recipe so that you will know exactly what you are putting in your body.

There are plenty of books on this subject on the market, so thanks again for choosing this one! Every effort was made to ensure it is full of as much useful information as possible. Please enjoy!

Chapter 1: Is Weight Loss Surgery Right for You?

Gastric sleeve surgeries are some of the most life-changing medical procedures a person can go through. The results are often dramatic weight loss and a decrease in health risks. Of course, this type of surgery is a better choice for some people than it is for others. How do you know if you could be a potential candidate for weight loss surgery? The rest of this chapter will provide details about whether bariatric weight loss surgery may be a good option for you.

Guidelines

In order to be considered as a candidate for gastric bypass surgeries, you generally need to have already exhausted other methods for losing weight. Your doctor will most likely ask you about your typical diet, as well as diets and exercises that you have tried in the past. He or she will also need information about your current exercise routine. Your general health and risks of obesity-related health issues will be taken into account as well. In most cases, your BMI (body mass index) must be at least 40 in order to be a candidate for surgery. Sometimes, people who have a BMI of at least 35 are considered. Typically, with the lower BMI of 35, you also have obesity-related severe medical issues such as type 2 diabetes or persistent high blood pressure.

In addition to these guidelines, you will go through the screening processes to determine if weight loss surgery is the best option for you as an individual. The medical team wants to be sure that the surgery will be beneficial to you and that the risks are outweighed by the benefits. Other factors that the medical team will look at are your psychiatric profile, your age, and the level of motivation that you show to become a healthier person with the assistance of bariatric surgery. Surgeries can be performed on teenagers if the benefits greatly outweigh the risks. Bariatric surgeries have also been performed on people who are aged 60 years and over if the benefits are greater than the risks associated with surgery and anesthesia. Prior to surgery, you may be required to show proof that you have made changes to your lifestyle in terms of diet and exercise in preparation for life after your gastric sleeve surgery.

Are you ready for surgery?

Aside from the medical perspective on things, you will have many other questions to ask yourself before deciding if you are ready to go through with a life-altering surgical procedure. You will need to determine how to pay for the procedure. If you have health insurance, you must first receive a pre-approval in order to know what will be covered by the insurance company, and what, if any, portion of the expenses you will be required to cover.

You also have to understand that the surgery itself is not a magical solution. It is only one of the many tools you will use to reach your goal of a healthier lifestyle at a lower weight. In order to reach your full potential after surgery, you will need to be dedicated to a healthier lifestyle. You will have to make nutritional changes to your diet, and you have to start exercising regularly or increase exercise if you are already active. There is also a high probability that you will need to take multivitamins and other supplements, as bariatric surgeries inhibit your body's ability to absorb nutrients.

There are some other points to consider when questioning bariatric surgery for weight loss. People who have struggled with alcohol or medicinal addiction in the past may not be good candidates for gastric bypass surgeries. Similarly, cigarette smokers will need to quit smoking many months before surgery. You will be required to enroll in educational classes before your surgery. Some of these classes will be for you to learn about proper nutrition. This means that you must be able to make time to attend the classes. Some of the screenings that you go through prior to scheduling a surgery may include imaging studies that will monitor your digestive system, as well as blood tests.

Risks associated with surgery

All surgeries have risks that are associated with them that may occur during or after surgery. Weight loss surgeries are no different, and your medical team will help you to measure the benefits and the risks. You will most likely have low levels of calcium, iron, vitamins, and minerals after surgery. This issue can be easily prevented or solved by the addition of daily multivitamins and other necessary supplements. You may experience something called dumping syndrome, which has symptoms of nausea, vomiting, diarrhea, and abdominal cramping. Your intestines may narrow in the areas in which surgery was performed. These narrowed areas are called strictures. If you do not follow recommendations, you may not lose weight or may gain weight back after it is lost. You may also develop a need for another related surgery. Speaking with your doctor will help you determine if you may be a good candidate and if the timing is right for you to undergo a surgery.

Key Points

- Weight loss surgeries are life-changing procedures.

- Surgery in and of itself is not a solution. It is merely a tool that you use in attaining weight loss and a healthier lifestyle.

- You will need to change your eating habits and exercise habits to benefit from surgery.

- You must go through the screening processes to determine if you are a good candidate and which type of surgery will be most beneficial to you.

- The screening processes may include blood testing and imaging sessions.

- You should also consider the financial aspects of surgery, as it can be quite expensive and may or may not be covered by health insurance.

- You will be required to attend educational sessions prior to your surgery to learn about proper nutrition, among other learning opportunities.

- There are risks associated with bariatric surgeries, as with all surgeries. Your doctor will help you determine if the benefits are greater than the associated risks.

Chapter 2: Types of Gastric Sleeve Surgeries

There are four types of gastric bypass surgeries that are among the most commonly performed for weight loss purposes. Each of these kinds of surgeries has associated positive and negative components. There are similarities and differences between the various surgery choices. The four types will be explained below.

It is important to remember that all types of gastric bypass surgery will require changes in diet and exercise in order to reduce health risks and to be successful. You may need to begin taking a daily multivitamin or other supplements due to nutrient absorption issues. You will have the best and healthiest results by working closely with your doctor or surgeon to decide which surgery is right for you, and what your postoperative lifestyle should be like.

Sleeve Gastrectomy

Sleeve gastrectomy limits the size of the stomach by removing a part of it laparoscopically. It works by affecting the amount of food that can be consumed. As a result of the surgery, the hormones are also affected and will assist in the process of losing weight. A benefit is that the hormonal changes can also trigger changes in blood pressure, which will help prevent heart disease. Approximately 80 percent of the stomach is cut away during the surgery, and the organ is left in a tubular shape. The new functional stomach is much smaller than before surgery. Since this is the case, much smaller food portions will be eaten, reducing the overall caloric intake. This option is typically available for people who have a BMI (body mass index) of at least 40. Having this surgery can help you to lose weight and reduce your risk of life-threatening health issues caused by obesity. (Mayo Clinic, n.d.)

Duodenal Switch with Biliopancreatic Diversion

This surgery has two parts. The first part is similar to a sleeve gastrectomy, which removes approximately 80 percent of the stomach. The difference in this surgery is that the pyloric valve that releases food from the stomach is not removed, nor is the duodenum. These two parts will remain in the body. The duodenum is the part of the intestines to which the stomach connects. The second part of this surgery connects the end portion of the intestines to the duodenum. This will cause a reduction in the amount of food that you can consume. It also causes a reduction in the number of nutrients that can be absorbed by the body.

As with sleeve gastrectomy, the new stomach is much smaller, this causes smaller portions to be ingested. The use of less of the intestines contributes to weight loss by reducing the overall absorption of nutrients. The majority of nutrients pass through the digestive system before they are effectively absorbed. This type of surgery is less common than sleeve gastrectomy. It is reserved for people with a BMI of at least 50. The surgery can only be an option if you have already unsuccessfully tried diet and exercise changes to attempt weight loss. It will help you to lose weight and lessen your risk of obesity-related health concerns. (Mayo Clinic, n.d.)

Laparoscopic Adjustable Gastric Banding

The stomach's top section is wrapped around in an adjustable band in this type of surgery. Only a small pouch of the former stomach will remain functional, allowing you to eat less and lose weight. There will be a port placed under your abdominal skin that will allow for the band to adjust. Adjustments are made to the fluid content of a balloon that has been placed under the band. Your doctor can make these changes at appointments, by inserting a needle into the port to add or decrease the amount of fluid that the balloon holds. As with the prior two surgeries, this one also is effective because the functioning amount of the stomach is much smaller. The biggest difference is that the amount of stomach that is portioned off can be adjusted after the surgery is complete. This choice is best for people with a BMI between 40 and 50. If your BMI is over 50, you may not lose as much weight as you desire with this option. (John Hopkins Medicine Health Library, n.d.)

Roux-En-Y Gastric Bypass

This is somewhat the same with the gastric banding but does not specifically use a sleeve or band. It is included here for comparison purposes because it is a common type of bariatric surgery and it also ultimately reduces the size of the stomach. The upper portion of the stomach is stapled off. The result is a pouch that is the size of a chicken egg. The new pouch is attached directly to the intestines, creating a "y" shape. This surgery will help you lose weight by reducing the number of calories and fat that you absorb from foods, along with a reduction in the absorption of minerals and vitamins. After having this surgery, you will be on a modified diet. It will be approximately one-month post surgery before you are able to return to eating normal foods. This option is best for people with a BMI of at least 40. (John Hopkins Medicine Health Library, n.d.)

Key Points

- All gastric sleeve surgeries have risks and benefits associated with them.

- There are similarities that are common factors in the surgeries that are offered, but each surgery has its own sets of positive and negative aspects.

- Most gastric bypass surgeries are performed laparoscopically.

- The duodenal switch with biliopancreatic diversion is ideal for people with a BMI of at least 50. The rest of the commonly performed gastric banding surgeries are ideal for those with a BMI of at least 40.

- Roux-en-Y gastric bypass surgery and duodenal switch with biliopancreatic diversion surgery reduce the absorption of nutrients.

- Laparoscopic adjustable gastric banding allows for adjustments to stomach size to be made by your doctor. You will also be left with a port after surgery so that the adjustments can be completed.

- Discussion with your doctor will help you to determine which surgical choice is best for you.

Chapter 3: The Recovery Phase

Following gastric sleeve surgery, your life will likely look much different than before you started your process as a candidate for the procedure. You will have to take especially good care of yourself and attend all post-op appointments. You will also learn to eat nutritiously with a smaller stomach and developing new exercise routines.

Post-Operative Care

You may spend the first one or two days after surgery in the hospital. This is an excellent time to review any question you might have with your doctor. You might want to go over things such as pain medications, returning to your normal activities, and care for your surgical incision.

You should let your doctor know immediately if you experience any symptoms that could be a result of your surgery. These include a fever, difficulty in breathing, abdominal pain, vomiting, diarrhea, or an incision that feels hot or painful. These could also be signs of infection.

For the first couple of weeks following surgery, you will probably only be permitted to consume a liquid diet. Once you begin to eat regular foods, you must remember to eat slowly while chewing your food well. You will also need to refrain from drinking for a half hour before you eat and for one-half hour after eating.

Nutritional absorption issues may develop after a bariatric surgery. Your doctor will help you to prevent this by telling you to take multivitamins and supplements each day. In addition to a general multivitamin, you may be advised to also take calcium and iron supplements, as well as vitamins D and B12. For the rest of your life, you will most likely take blood tests twice yearly to ascertain your nutritional levels and to determine if any changes should be made to the supplements that you take.

Foods That Promote Recovery and Healing

Some foods are healthier choices than others. After undergoing a weight loss procedure, it is very important to opt for nutrient dense foods that will meet the needs of your diet. There are some foods that are especially noted for their restorative and healing properties such as foods that are high in antioxidants and vitamins. Foods that are rich in vitamins A, C, and D are especially beneficial in aiding healing after surgery. Foods with high levels of vitamin A include dark green vegetables like kale and spinach and orange vegetables like sweet potatoes and carrots. Berries, oranges, melons, tomatoes, and bell peppers are all vitamin C rich. Vitamin D can be found in fish, eggs, milk, and some cereals. Grapes, pomegranates, and all types of berries are full of antioxidants. Antioxidant repair damage to the body. Healthy fats such as nuts, avocado, and olive oil can help your body absorb the vitamins it needs to heal properly. Other highly nutritious foods to ensure you are eating include bok choy, seafood, eggs, beans, and whole grains. Bok choy can contribute to your vitamin K intake, seafood and eggs deliver protein, and beans and whole grains will keep your energy levels up. Yogurt will provide healthy probiotics that will help you with digestion.

Getting In and Staying In Shape with Exercise

Getting proper nutrition is only half the battle in gaining a new healthier lifestyle after weight loss surgery. You will also need to determine what types of exercise will benefit you most and develop a workout routine. You will likely combine some sort of cardio and weight training activities. Always discuss with your medical team to ascertain a safe time to begin adding workouts to your schedule.

Swimming, cycling, and walking are generally the best places to start for low-intensity cardio or aerobic exercises. You will slowly increase your daily activity to add in a stroll through the park, or using the stairs instead of an elevator. Once you get started, you will have an eventual goal of 60 minutes of moderate exercise. Low-intensity exercise is best for weight loss. You will want to exercise on most days, but it is important to take approximately one day a week off to allow your body to rest and make any needed repairs. If you ever feel joint pain, that is not a typical result, and you should make alterations to your exercising routine. The majority of exercise that you do should be of the cardio or aerobic variety, but it is good to add in about 15 minutes of weight training or strength training as well.

Weight training or strength training is fine to add to your workouts up to three times each week. However, you will want to make sure that you space the sessions out by a minimum of 48 hours. Start off slow with light weights and build up as you progress. It is better to have more repetitions than heavier weights to reach a weight loss goal. Lastly, make sure that you are switching up your workouts every six weeks or so. Your body can become complacent with the same exercise routine for long periods of time, so changes are needed to keep your weight loss going.

Key Points

- After your surgery, you will most likely have a short hospital stay.
- Consult with your doctor for the answers to any questions that you may have.
- Be on the lookout for any symptoms of infection.
- Difficulty in the absorption of nutrients is a known side effect of bariatric procedures.
- Nutritional supplements and multivitamins can help to offset difficulty in absorbing needed nutrients.
- Eat small, healthy portions of nutrient dense foods.
- Foods that are rich in protein, antioxidants, and vitamins will be the best for helping you heal after surgery.
- Probiotics are beneficial for digestion.
- Exercise when you have the go-ahead from your doctor.
- Add physical activity slowly.

- Start with light cardio activities and increase exercise until you have six days a week of 60-minute aerobic intervals.

- Adding in weight training or strength training can aid in losing weight and building lean muscle.

- Switch up workout routines often to continue losing weight.

Chapter 4: Recipes for Recovery

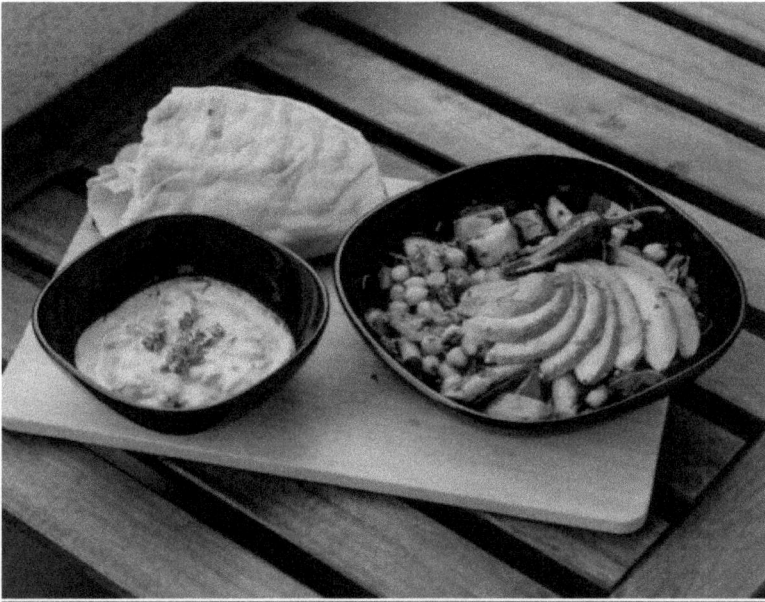

While recovering from gastric bypass surgery, you need to be assured that you are receiving adequate nutrients such as vitamins and protein. You will also be eating smaller portions than you are used to after obtaining a gastric sleeve. In order to recover healthfully, it is necessary to eat nutritious foods in variety.

The recipes contained within this book have all been developed especially for patients who have undergone gastric sleeve surgeries. In addition, these recipes contain ingredients that are known to promote healing and recovery and contain nutrition information at the end of each. The serving sizes are all small portions and the foods are delicious. You will find options for breakfasts, lunches, dinners, snacks, and even desserts. Start exploring and choose your favorites!

Egg Muffins

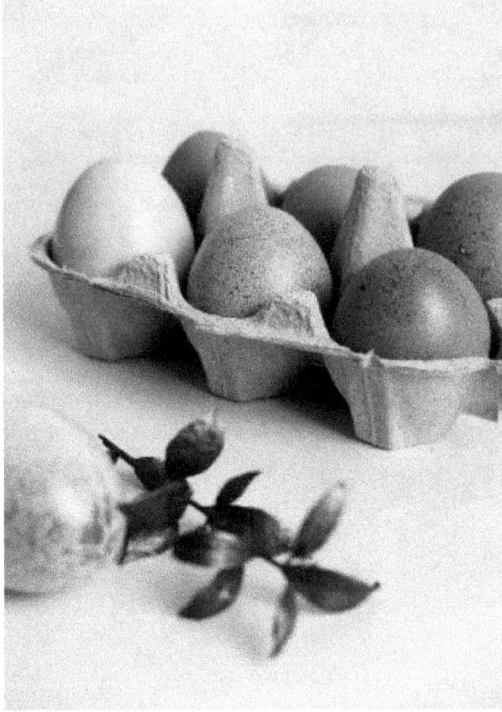

This delicious recipe can be prepped ahead for breakfast on-the-go. Eggs and turkey bacon provide protein to promote healing.

Ingredients:

- Black pepper, .25 teaspoons
- Salt, .25 teaspoons
- 1% milk, .5 c
- Shredded cheese, low fat, .75 c
- Turkey bacon, precooked, 12 slices
- Eggs, 6 large

Preparation Method:

1. Set your oven to 350 degrees.
2. Put one crumbled bacon slice at the bottom of one of the muffin cups of a muffin tin.
3. Except for the cheese, mix all of the other ingredients together.
4. Put .25 c of the mixture in each muffin cup.
5. Sprinkle the shredded cheese over the tops of the muffins.
6. Bake the egg muffins for 20 to 25 minutes.

Number of servings: 12

Size of serving: 1 muffin

- 98 calories
- 7 grams fat
- 2 grams saturated fat
- 1 gram carbohydrates
- 0 gram fiber
- 1 gram sugar
- 8 grams protein

Breakfast Berry Wrap

Berries provide antioxidants needed for healing and whole grains for energy. This breakfast can be prepared quickly and easily, no baking required.

Ingredients:

- Sliced strawberries, fresh, .25 c
- Strawberry jelly, low sugar, 1 Tablespoon
- Ricotta cheese, 3 Tablespoons
- Whole wheat tortilla, 1

Preparation Method:

1. Spread the jelly and the ricotta cheese on the tortilla.
2. Sprinkle the strawberries.
3. Roll the tortilla up and serve.

Serving size: 1 wrap

Number of servings: 1

- 229 milligrams sodium
- 233 calories
- 24 milligrams cholesterol
- 30 grams carbohydrates
- 9 grams fat
- 8 grams sugar
- 8 grams protein

Black Bean and Corn Salad

A delightful mixture of beans and corn will provide protein and energy. There is no cooking necessary, so this recipe is easy enough for anyone to try out.

Ingredients:

- Whole kernel corn, 1 cup
- Lemon juice, 1 teaspoon
- Minced garlic, 1 teaspoon
- Olive oil, 2 Tablespoons
- Honey, 1 teaspoon
- Black pepper, .25 teaspoons
- Minced red onion, 2 Tablespoons
- Balsamic vinegar, .25 cups
- Drained and rinsed black beans, (2) 16 oz cans
- Fresh parsley, .25 cups

Preparation Method:

1. Mix the corn, black beans, red onion, and pepper in a large mixing dish.
2. All of the other ingredients should be whisked.
3. Pour the liquids over the mixture.
4. Marinate the salad for 30 minutes before serving.

Serving size: .25 c

Number of servings: 6

- 306 milligrams potassium
- 40 milligrams sodium
- 0 milligram cholesterol
- 6 grams protein
- 3 grams sugar
- 6 grams fiber
- 23 grams g carbohydrates
- 5 grams fat
- 160 calories

Baked Chicken and Vegetables

A classic dinner takes on a new life in this recipe. Cook dinner for the family or meal prep and have this recipe for lunches and dinners. Protein and vitamin A will aid in the recovery.

Ingredients:

- Black pepper, .25 t
- Thyme, 1 teaspoon
- Water, .5 c
- Raw skinless chicken, 1
- Quartered onion, 1 large
- Sliced carrots, 6
- Sliced potatoes, 4

Preparation Method:

1. Preheat your oven to 400 degrees.
2. Put the carrots, potatoes, and onions in a large oven-safe dish.
3. Place the chicken over the vegetables.
4. Mix up the water, black pepper, and thyme.
5. Pour this mixture over the vegetables and chicken.
6. Spoon the cooking juices over the chicken two times while cooking. Bake for at least one hour until the chicken is browned.

Serving size: one-sixth of the recipe

Number of servings: 6

- 130 milligram sodium

- 26 grams protein

- 10 grams sugar

- 4grams fiber

- 25 gram carbohydrates

- 3.5 gram fat

- 240 calories

Asian Style Lettuce Wraps

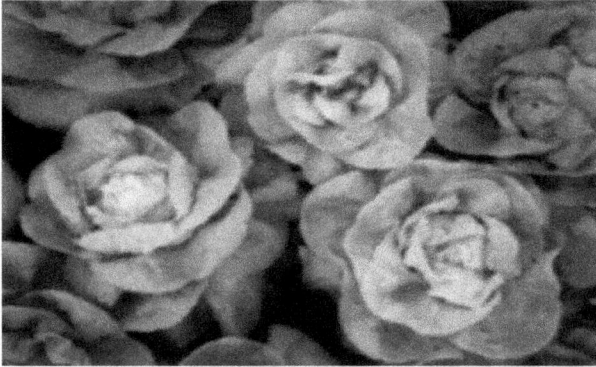

Full of flavor, this recipe provides you with plenty of protein! This one is great for a group or as a make-ahead meal.

Ingredients:

- Sliced cucumber, 1 small
- Chopped green onion, 1 whole
- Butter lettuce, 8 leaves
- Sesame oil, toasted, 1 teaspoon
- Minced ginger, 1 teaspoon
- Ground chicken breast, .5 lb
- Minced onion, 1 c
- Minced garlic, 1 Tablespoon
- Splenda, 2 packets
- Sriracha hot sauce, 2 teaspoon
- Peanut butter, unsalted, 1 Tablespoon
- Soy sauce, low sodium, 2 teaspoons
- Hoisin sauce, 2 Tablespoons

Preparation Method:

1. Combine hoisin sauce, sriracha, peanut butter, soy sauce, and Splenda in a bowl and mix well.

2. Place a nonstick skillet over medium heat.

3. Cook the onion for four minutes. Mix in the garlic and cook for one more minute.

4. Add the ground chicken and ginger.

5. Increase the temperature of the burner to medium-high heat.

6. Break the chicken up and cook it until there is no pink color left.

7. Stir the sesame oil in and remove from the heat.

8. Divide the product evenly among the lettuce leaves.

9. Top with cucumber and green onion.

Serving size: 2 wraps

Number of servings: 4

- 637 milligrams sodium
- 33 milligrams cholesterol
- 16 grams protein
- 4 grams sugar
- 5 grams fiber
- 11 grams carbohydrates
- 4 grams fat
- 155 calories

Cheesesteak Wrap

Yes, you can still enjoy a chicken cheesesteak. With a few tweaks to the original, this recipe contains protein, vitamin C, and antioxidants.

Ingredients:

- Low carb tortilla, 1
- Light Swiss cheese, .75 oz
- Sliced mushrooms, .25 c
- Sliced green peppers, .25 c
- Chopped onions, .25 c
- Skinless, boneless chicken breast, .25 lb

Preparation Method:

1. Pound the chicken breast until it is .25 inch thin. Then create thin strips by cutting it with a knife.
2. Cook the chicken on the medium-high heat in a cooking pan with the onions.
3. Add the mushrooms and the green pepper and continue cooking.
4. Warm the tortilla for 20 seconds in the microwave, then place in the middle of two damp paper towels.
5. Spread the cheese in the middle of the tortilla.
6. Add the vegetables and the chicken.
7. Fold up the tortilla and serve.

Serving size: 1 wrap

Number of servings: 1

- 620 milligrams sodium

- 76 milligrams cholesterol

- 3 grams protein

- 4 grams fiber

- 264 calories

- 17 grams carbohydrates

- 6 grams fat

Beef Ginger Stir Fry

Instead of going out, try to make a stir-fry for you at home. This recipe provides plenty of protein, vitamin A, and whole grains for energy.

Ingredients:

- Water chestnuts, 8 oz
- Bok choy, 2 medium stalks, cut in .5 inch slices
- Brown rice, instant, .5 c
- Medium bell pepper, .5 cut in strips
- Broccoli florets, 3 oz
- Red pepper flakes, crushed, .25 teaspoons
- Soy sauce, 3 Tablespoons
- Cornstarch, 1 Tablespoon
- Canola oil, 1 teaspoon
- Beef broth, 6 oz fat-free
- Garlic cloves, 2 medium
- Ground ginger, 2 teaspoon
- Flank steak, 1 lb (in .25 inch strips)

Preparation Method:

1. Mix the garlic, ginger, and steak slices in a bowl and set it aside.
2. Stir the broth, soy sauce, and cornstarch together in a separate bowl.

3. Heat the oil in a skillet over medium-high heat. Add the pepper flakes.

4. Constantly stir the steak while cooking it for four to five minutes, and then set it aside.

5. Cook the bell pepper and broccoli for two to three minutes. Then add the water chestnuts and the bok choy.

6. In the center of the pan, make a well to put in the broth.

7. Cook this for one to two minutes, and then mix the beef in and cook for an additional one to two minutes.

8. Serve the stir-fry over the rice.

Serving size: .25 of the total

Number of servings: 4

- 17 grams protein
- 6 grams sugar
- 2 grams fiber
- 25 grams carbohydrates
- 8 grams fat
- 275 calories

Zucchini Boats

Chock full of antioxidants and protein, this recipe will assist in healing. It makes many servings, so this is a good recipe for making ahead or for a family dinner.

Ingredients:

- Low-fat shredded mozzarella cheese, 1 c
- Black pepper, .25 t
- Whole wheat bread crumbs, .25 c
- Spaghetti sauce, .75 c
- Diced tomato, 1 large
- Sliced mushrooms, .5 lb
- Beaten egg, 1
- Chopped onion, .5 c
- Ground turkey, 1 lb
- Zucchini, 4 medium

Preparation Method:

1. Slice the zucchinis lengthwise in half. Scoop out the pulp to create boats and set it aside.
2. Put the boats in a large dish safe for use in the microwave. Cover the dish, and then heat it in the microwave for three minutes on high.
3. In a skillet, cook the onion and turkey on the medium-high heat.

4. Drain the turkey mix.

5. Mix the zucchini pulp, egg, bread crumbs, spaghetti sauce, tomato, mushrooms, cheese, pepper, and turkey mix.

6. Place a quarter cup of the mix into each one of the shells.

7. Bake for 20 minutes, uncovered, at 350 degrees.

Serving size: 1 boat

Number of servings: 8

- 294 milligrams sodium
- 17.5 grams protein
- 5 grams sugar
- 4 grams fiber
- 16 grams carbohydrates
- 7.5 grams fat
- 195 calories

Veggie Pizza

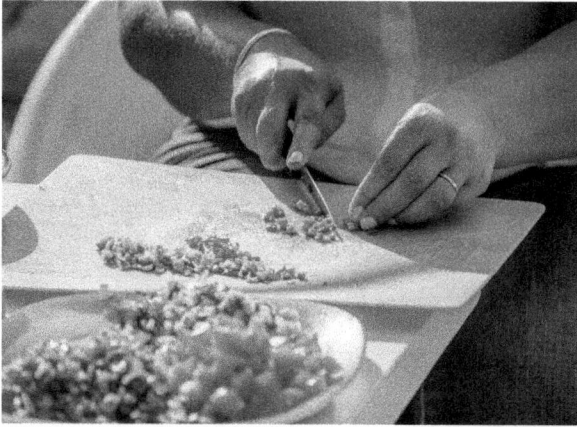

This recipe is fun for parties or an evening at home. Plenty of vegetables make it great for recovery and healing.

Ingredients:

- Black olives, .5 c sliced
- Shredded Colby jack cheese, low fat .75c
- Diced cucumbers, .25 c
- Diced green pepper, .25 c
- Diced tomatoes, .25 c
- Diced broccoli, raw .75 c
- Shredded carrots, .25 c
- Ranch dressing dry mix, 1 package
- Sour cream, low fat, .5 c
- Cream cheese, low fat, .5c
- Large low carb wraps 2

Preparation Method:

1. Mix the ranch dry mix, sour cream, and cream cheese until combined.
2. Spread the ranch combination on the tortillas.
3. Use the vegetables as toppings.
4. Sprinkle the cheese over the top.
5. Divide the tortillas into quarters and serve.

Serving size: .25 tortilla

Number of servings: 8

- 870 milligrams sodium
- 23 milligrams cholesterol
- 10 grams protein
- 1.6 grams sugar
- 4 grams fiber
- 12 grams carbohydrates
- 10 grams fat
- 170 calories

Hummus

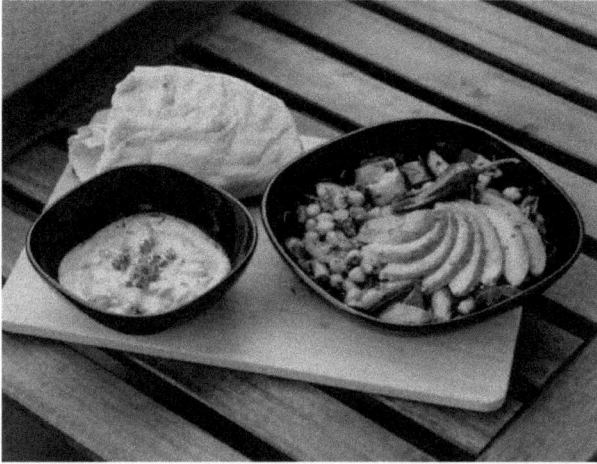

This is a classic hummus recipe. Use it for a vegetable dip or for salads.

Ingredients:

- Salt, .5 teaspoon
- Chickpeas, (1) 15 oz can rinsed
- Lemon juice, 3 Tablespoons
- Olive oil, 3 Tablespoons
- Tahini, 1 Tablespoon
- Garlic, clove 1 peeled

Preparation Method:

1. Chop the garlic in a food processor.
2. Add all of the other listed ingredients.
3. Blend the ingredients one to two minutes, until entirely smooth.

Serving size: 2

Number of servings: 12

- 149 milligrams sodium
- 0 milligram cholesterol
- 6 grams protein
- 0 gram sugar
- 72 calories
- 7.5 grams carbohydrates
- 4.5 grams fat

Spicy Devilled Eggs

This is a great snack to have on hand for a little protein. You can make it ahead and have it ready.

Ingredients:

- Paprika a dash
- Black pepper a dash
- Hard boiled eggs, 6 whites, 3 yolks
- Dijon mustard .25 t
- Dill .5 t
- Greek yogurt 2 T

Preparation Method:

1. Peel all of the eggs and slice them lengthwise in half.
2. Set aside the whites. Put three yolks in a bowl to mix.
3. Mash the yolks with the yogurt, dijon, and dill.
4. Spoon the filling in the half eggs.
5. Sprinkle paprika and black pepper on the tops of the eggs.

Serving size: 2 egg halves

Number of servings: 3

- 219 milligrams sodium
- 225 milligrams cholesterol

- 10 grams protein
- 0 gram sugar
- 131 calories
- 1 gram carbohydrates
- 8.7 grams fat

Soy Chocolate Dessert

This is a recipe for a pudding made with tofu. The tofu makes the dessert creamy and healthy, and the protein helps you heal.

Ingredients:

- Vanilla extract, .5 t
- Silken tofu, 16 oz
- Skim milk, 1 c
- Fat-free, sugar-free chocolate fudge pudding, instant, 1 package
- Hot water, .25 c
- Unflavored gelatin, 1 envelope

Preparation Method:

1. Mix the hot water and gelatin in a small bowl and allow it to set.
2. Dice the tofu in one-inch cubes and put it in a mixing bowl with the pudding.
3. Add vanilla extract and place the mixture in a blender.
4. Blend until you reach a smooth texture, and then add the gelatin gradually until well-combined. Blend once more.
5. Pour the mix in an 8-inch by 8-inch dish.
6. Cover and leave the dish in the refrigerator for at least 30 minutes.

Serving size: .5 c

Number of servings: 8

- 181 milligrams sodium
- 1 milligram cholesterol
- 5 grams protein
- 6 grams carbohydrates
- 1 grams fat
- 56 calories

Cheesecake Pudding

Here is a dessert that takes no time at all to make. Greek yogurt provides protein that is needed for the healing process.

Ingredients:

- Cheesecake flavored pudding mix 1 packet, sugar-free
- Greek yogurt 1 c, plain, fat-free

Preparation Method:

1. In a blender, puree the ingredients until they are combined.

Serving size: .5 c

Number of servings: 2

- 7 grams protein
- 4.5 grams sugar
- 3 grams carbohydrates
- 0 grams fat
- 62 calories

PART 3

ACKNOWLEDGMENTS

We would like to acknowledge the American Thyroid Association and the hard work of everyone involved in the prevention and treatment of any and all thyroid conditions, which affect the health and lives of many loved ones. Thank you.

Introduction

The reasons to pick up a book of this sort are many. Perhaps you have picked this title because you are currently suffering from an issue with your thyroid gland. Maybe you have in the past and wish to get a greater understanding of what it was that you went through. Or you may even just want to be prepared for the eventuality and desire the knowledge necessary to prevent an issue with the thyroid gland of yourself or your loved ones from occurring altogether.

Whatever your reasons, whatever it is you are seeking to gain from choosing this text, it will provide you with the answers and with needed help. For it is easy to overlook or not keep in mind the thyroid gland despite its importance and role in the maintenance of our health.

Conditions afflicting the thyroid gland are in no way scarce and can be made to become quite severe, if and when left unattended to in the proper manner, or by the proper medical authorities. With that in mind do not worry, there is no need to feel intimidated or overly cautious about diving into this subject matter. You have already taken the correct first steps in supplementing and elevating the health of your thyroid gland. You have picked up this title and chosen to become more informed and play a more active role when it comes to the health of your thyroid gland, yourself and your body.

Thank you for doing so, and please enjoy.

Chapter 1: What in The World Is A Thyroid

In this chapter, we will be exploring just what the thyroid is, and its functions in maintaining and keeping your body healthy.

For starters, the word thyroid has its origins dating as far back as the 1690s. Coming from the Greek, *thyreoiedes*, meaning "shield-shaped". Also referred to as, *khondros thyreoiedes*, "shield-shaped cartilage". Aptly named, as the thyroid gland is an organ which is often considered to resemble a butterfly, bow tie, or shield shape, at the base of the neck.

The thyroid gland plays an extremely vital role in the way your body uses energy, by releasing hormones that aid in controlling your body's metabolism. The hormones released by the thyroid gland assist in regulating important body functions, including but not limited to:

- Regulation of breathing
- Heart rate
- The central and peripheral nervous systems
- Body weight
- Cycles of menstruation
- The strength of muscles
- Levels of cholesterol
- The temperature of the body

Quite a lot for an organ coming in at only around 2 inches long. This tiny but important gland rests in the front portion of the throat, in front of the trachea, and just below the thyroid cartilage commonly referred to as the

Adam's apple. The Adam's apple itself is the largest cartilage of the voice box or larynx.

Owing to the bow tie, butterfly, or shield shape, of the thyroid gland, is a middle connection of thin thyroid tissue, which is known as the isthmus, which is responsible for holding together two lobes on the right and left sides of it. It is not entirely uncommon, however, for someone to be missing the isthmus all-together and instead of having the two lobes of the thyroid gland operating separate from one another.

Now that you are aware of this and may feel a bit more familiar with your own thyroid gland, you may resist trying to see or feel around for it in your neck yourself. Unless the thyroid gland is otherwise afflicted and made to become enlarged, mostly known as a goiter, the thyroid will be unable to be seen, and only just barely able to be felt. It is only when a goiter occurs and the neck is swollen from an enlarged thyroid that it will be at all noticeable either to the eye or to the touch.

The thyroid gland is one of the major players in the endocrine system. The endocrine system includes glands that are responsible for the production and for the secretion of various hormones. The other organs which help make up the endocrine system are the hypothalamus, which is responsible for linking the body's nervous system to the endocrine system via the use of the pituitary gland. The pituitary gland which is responsible for the secretion of hormones, not the blood stream. The pineal gland, which produces the wake/sleep pattern hormone of melatonin. The adrenal glands, which are responsible for the production of a variety of hormones like the steroids cortisol and aldosterone as well as our body's adrenaline.

The Pancreas, an organ located in the abdominal region of the body, the primary role of which is the converting of food into fuel for the body's cells. The ovaries and testicles, sex organs of the body. And the parathyroid glands.

Utilizing the iodine content from foods, the thyroid is able to produce and churn out the hormones T3, which stands for triiodothyronine, and the hormone T4, thyroxine.

T3, or triiodothyronine, is merely the active form of the companion hormone thyroxine, or T4. The thyroid gland alone is able to secrete around 20% of our body's T3 into the bloodstream on its own. With the other 80% coming from organs like the liver and the kidneys going through the process of converting thyroxine into its active counterpart.

It is absolutely possible for your body to have far too much of T3 though. When there is an over secretion of T3 into the blood stream, it is called thyrotoxicosis. This can be due to a number of conditions dealing with the thyroid gland such as overactivity in the thyroid gland, known as hyperthyroidism, caused by such conditions as a benign tumor, the thyroid gland becoming enflamed, or a condition known as graves' disease. The previously mentioned condition of a goiter, in which the neck begins to swell, might be a signal of thyrotoxicosis having occurred. Even more symptoms to have an eye out for in case of hyperthyroidism will be an increase in the appetite, increased regularity of bowel movements, an intolerance to heat, the loss of weight, the menstrual cycle becoming irregulated, a heartbeat becoming increasingly rapid or irregular in rhythm, the thinning or loss of hair, tremors, becoming irritable, overly tired, palpitations, and the eyelids retracting.

It is also possible for your body to be producing too little of the hormone T3. The thyroid gland producing too little of T3 is known commonly as hypothyroidism. It is common for autoimmune diseases to have a strong role in this occurring, an example of which would be the Hashimoto's disease, which causes the immune system to attack the thyroid gland. Certain medications or the intake of too little iodine can also cause hypothyroidism. This can be very serious, especially if a case of hypothyroidism goes unnoticed or untreated during early childhood, or even before birth. With the regulation of hormones being so important, primarily to physical and mental development, not treating hypothyroidism during these crucial times often result in reduced growth for the child, or becoming learning disabled.

The affliction of hypothyroidism is not foreign to adults though. When hypothyroidism occurs in adults they tend to have the functions of their bodies slowed down drastically. The effects of hypothyroidism in an adult have been known to include symptoms such as a growing intolerance to colder temperature, the heart rate of the adult will lower, gaining weight, a reduction in appetite, the ability of memory becomes poorer, fertility will reduce, muscles will become stiff, the adult may become depressed, and tired.

T4, or thyroxine, is the primary hormone that gets secreted from the thyroid gland and into the body's bloodstream. Unlike T3 which is active, thyroxine is in an inactive form and most of it will need to be converted to the active form, triiodothyronine, which is a process that takes place in organs like the kidneys and liver. Undergoing these processes is vital in making sure the body is able to regulate a healthy metabolic rate, control of the body's muscles, development of the brain, develop and maintain bones, and digestive and heart functionality.

As with T3, triiodothyronine, the production and secretion of too much will inevitable result in thyrotoxicosis, while the production and secretion of too little thyroxine, will result in hypothyroidism.

To combat this, the body and thyroid gland have a few tricks vital to the regulation of levels of these hormones in the cells. There is a controlled feedback loop system, involving the hypothalamus in the brain as well as in the thyroid gland and pituitary gland which is in control of the production of both of the hormones thyroxine and triiodothyronine. Thyrotropin-releasing hormones are secreted from the hypothalamus and, in turn, the pituitary gland becomes stimulated into producing thyroid stimulating hormone. A hormone which will stimulate thyroxine and triiodothyronine to be produced and secreted by the thyroid gland.

A feedback loop regulates this production system, to account for the levels of thyroxine and of triiodothyronine. If the levels of either of these thyroid gland hormones begin to increase, they will end up preventing the production and secretion of the thyrotropin-releasing hormone as well as the thyroid stimulating hormone, thus allowing the body to maintain, on it's own, a steady level of the thyroid hormones that it needs.

For all these reasons it is of vital importance that the levels of T3 and T4 being secreted thru-ought the body and its cells never get too high or too low. T3 and T4 are able to reach just about ever cell in the body by utilizing the bloodstream. The rate of work for the cells and metabolism to work is regulated by the hormones T3 and T4. To make sure that levels are never either too high or too low, this is why we have a thyroid gland.

The final hormone that the thyroid gland is responsible for the production of is the hormone calcitonin, CT, or thyrocalcitonin. Within the thyroid gland are what are known as C-cells, or parafollicular cells, which are in charge of the proliferation of this particular hormone. The primary role of calcitonin in the body is to help in the regulation of the levels of phosphate in the blood, and of calcium in the blood. Doing so is to be in opposition of the parathyroid hormone. In short, meaning that what it aims to do is reduce the amount of calcium in the blood stream. The reason for playing this role in the human anatomy game has been a bit of a mystery to science up to this point though, due to the observation of patients showing either very high or even very low levels of the hormone calcitonin, having no adverse effect on them.

The hormone calcitonin has two primary mechanisms by which to aid in the reduction of calcium levels within the human body. It can completely inhibit the activity of the cells in our body which are responsible for breaking down bones, known as osteoclasts. Osteoclasts do this because when bone is broken down, the calcium within the bone being broken down will be released into the body's bloodstream. So by inhibiting the osteoclasts from doing their respective jobs, calcitonin is directly involved in the reduction of the amount of calcium that is getting released into the body's bloodstream. Despite doing this though, the length of time that calcitonin can cause this inhibition has been shown to be quite short. Calcitonin can be an active player in the resorption of calcium into the kidneys, which it does by lower the levels of blood calcium in the body.

Calcitonin has been manufactured in the past and has then been given, in this form, to treat the disease of bone, Paget's disease. Also known as osteitis deformans, Paget's disease is rather common, and is a chronic bone disorder which can cause pain, fractures or deformities of a bone, or show absolutely no symptoms at all. It is however easily able to be controlled and treated with proper early enough diagnosis and treatment.

The manufactured hormone calcitonin has also been given to sufferers of general bone pain, and of hypercalcaemia, which is when the body has an abnormal level of calcium flowing in the bloodstream.

Though because of the introduction of bisphosphonates, which aid in the preventing of the breakdown of bone cells and are drugs also used to help treat osteoporosis, the use of manufactured calcitonin has decreased.

Chapter 2: Possible Thyroid Disorders

In the previous chapter, we began to cover what it is exactly that the thyroid gland gets done and even dabbled a bit into how it does it's job properly. During the last chapter, we mentioned a few of the various thigs which can afflict the thyroid gland, why this may occur in certain circumstances, and what the effects of these afflictions could be. Moving on into chapter two is where we will begin to take a closer look at everything that can go wrong with the thyroid gland. Not just the what, but the why as well. What causes these changes in our thyroid gland to occur, and what to expect to happen when they do occur. The importance of having this knowledge be a part of your thyroid gland arsenal cannot be at all overstated as there is a wide array of severity to both the symptoms and to the results of the ailments that can afflict the thyroid gland and consequently hinder our body's ability to maintain its health properly.

Just as well in this chapter, you can expect to be reading deeper into some of the ailments that may have already been brought up in the previous chapter, such as hyperthyroidism, hypothyroidism, graves disease, goiters, and Hashimoto's disease.

Hyperthyroidism

As briefly discussed in the last chapter, hyperthyroidism is a rather common condition in which there is overactivity in the thyroid gland and begins to produce far too much of the thyroid hormone which would usually be used to regulate the body's metabolic rate. This can be an overproduction of the hormones T3, which is triiodothyronine, T4, which is tetraiodothyronine, or even an overproduction of both of these hormones.

The causes of hyperthyroidism can vary greatly, with the most common reason for it being the aforementioned Grave's disease, which we will go much further into later in the chapter. The basics of Grave's disease are that it is an autoimmune disorder which causes antibodies in the body to stimulate the thyroid gland making it secrete to many of it's hormones. You should tell your regular doctor if any one in your family has ever had Grave's disease as it seems to have a genetic link, being passed down commonly from generation to the next generation. Grave's disease is also known to be more prevalent in women, affecting about 1 percent of the female population, than it is in men.

Another common reason for hyperthyroidism to occur is an excess level of iodine in the body, which is the main ingredient in hormones T3 and T4.

Less common, but still just as relevant to the conversation as causes for hyperthyroidism is thyroiditis which is the inflammation of thyroid gland, which in turn will cause the hormones T3 and T4 to start leaking out of the thyroid gland.

Tumors located on the ovaries or testes have been known links to hyperthyroidism. As well as even tumors, even when benign, located on the thyroid gland, or pituitary gland.

An easily preventable cause of hyperthyroidism which should not be overlooked is the intake of large amounts of T4, or tetraiodothyronine, via the ingestion of a dietary supplement or of a prescribed medication.

When it comes to the symptoms of hyperthyroidism, believe it or not, we had only scratched the surface in the previous chapter and will be going more in-depth here on what you can expect to look out for in order to self-diagnose an issue before going to seek out a professional opinion.

To begin with, in the case of Grave's disease, one of the symptoms can be a bulging of the eyes as if stuck in a stare. Other symptoms to watch out for would be an increase in the appetite, perhaps an increase in nervousness or a sense of restlessness. Muscular weakness, the inability to concentrate on simple tasks, irregularity in the heartbeat, loss of the ability to sleep soundly or for long periods of time, the loss of hair, or noticing that your hair has become thinner or more brittle, can be signs of hyperthyroidism. Thinness of the skin is also common, as well as becoming more irritable, sweating more, or becoming more anxious. In men specifically, the development of breasts can be a sign of hyperthyroidism. And in women, hyperthyroidism has been known to have adverse effects on the regularity of the menstrual cycle.

If you experience any of the prior symptoms, it is, of course, recommended to seek out professional help and diagnosis. However, it is highly recommended that you seek out professional help for the treatment of hyperthyroidism if you begin to experience a sensation of dizziness if you start to notice shortness in your breathing, which will likely come with the increase in heart rate, making it faster and irregular, and any loss of consciousness. Having hyperthyroidism has also been known to be the cause of atrial fibrillations, which are a dangerous arrythmia, commonly responsible for leading to having a stroke, or even to congestive heart failures.

In diagnosing a case of hyperthyroidism, a doctor will likely begin the process by conducting a full and complete medical history, as well as a physical exam. These are commonly conducted as they are helpful in revealing the common signs of loss of weight, how rapid your pulse is, an elevation in pressure of the blood, protrusion of the eyes, or the enlargement of the thyroid gland itself.

It is also reasonable to expect your doctor to conduct a cholesterol test which will be done to check on the levels of cholesterol in your system. This is done because cholesterol levels being low can be an indication that there is an elevation in your metabolic rate, which would mean that your body is burning through your cholesterol far too quickly.

Doctors are also able to conduct tests to measure the levels of T3 and T4 that are in your blood. Thyroid stimulating hormone tests can be done to check the levels of TSH, or thyroid stimulating hormone coursing within your body. TSH stimulates your thyroid gland to produce the hormones the body needs, and if your thyroid gland is producing levels of hormones at a normal rate, or even a rate that is too high, your TSH should come out lower. And a level of TSH that is abnormally low can be an important signifier that you may have hyperthyroidism.

A triglyceride test will be done, because similarly to having low amounts of cholesterol, a low level of triglycerides can be significant of an elevation in your metabolic rate. A thyroid scan or uptake will allow a doctor to see if your thyroid gland is being overactive. It will actually get even more particular, and let a doctor be able to see if it is the entire thyroid gland which is acting up or just a particular area of the thyroid gland.

Ultrasounds have been known to be utilized, as they will allow a doctor to observe entirely, the size of the thyroid gland, as well as any masses that may be within the thyroid gland. It is the use of the ultrasound which will also be able to let the doctor know if the mass inside the thyroid gland is cystic, or if it is solid. Just as well a CT, Computed Tomography, or MRI, Magnetic Resonance Imaging, scan can be performed to show if the condition is being caused by a tumor being present on the pituitary gland.

Treatment of hyperthyroidism also comes in varieties and may be dependent on the cause of the hyperthyroidism. Perhaps the most common treatment comes in the form of medication. Generally an antithyroid medication like methimazole, also known as Tapazole, which will cause the thyroid gland to halt the production and secretion of hormones altogether.

According to the American Thyroid Association, around 70 percent of U.S. adults who undergo treatment for hyperthyroidism will receive a form of treatment called radioactive iodine. Radioactive iodine is essentially able to completely and effectively destroy the cells that would otherwise be producing hormones. Radioactive iodine, or RAI, in the form of a liquid or a pill, will be ingested by way of the mouth, and is safe to use on an individual who has had any allergic reaction to an X-ray contrast agent or to seafood, because essentially the reaction comes from the compound which contains iodine, and not from the iodine itself. The iodine, in an iodide form, is actually split into two forms or radioactive iodine, known as I-123, which is harmless to thyroid gland cells, and I-131, which is responsible for the destruction of thyroid gland cells. The radiation which is emitted by both of these forms of the iodine are able to be detected from outside of the patient, which will help the doctor to gain any information needed the thyroid glands functionality, and take any pictures needed of the size thyroid glands tissues, as well as their location in the body. This treatment is not without its side effects though, which generally tend to come in the presence of dryness of the mouth, soreness of the eyes and in the throat, and has also been known to effect changes in taste. You may also be required, if undergoing this treatment, to take precautions for a short time which will prevent the spread of radiation to others.

Surgery is yet another common form of treatment for hyperthyroidism. In this case, it is entirely possible that a section of your thyroid gland will be removed, though entire thyroid glands have also been removed in this procedure. This is followed up with taking thyroid hormone supplements which will help in the prevention of hypothyroidism, which is what happens when there is the occurrence of underactivity in the thyroid gland, causing it to produce and secrete too little of the intended hormones. Beta-blockers may also be taken, such as something like propranolol to help control a rapid pulse, sweating, any anxiety that may crop up, and higher blood pressure. It is reported that most people respond very well to this form of treatment.

If you would like to improve any symptoms, or even take action to prevent symptoms from occurring, you are not left without options. You can work along with your doctor, or a dietician, to help create a healthy guideline for diet, exercise, and any nutritional supplementation. Proper diet intake, with a stronger focus on getting calcium and sodium, can be crucially important in the prevention of hyperthyroidism. Osteoporosis is a common result of hyperthyroidism as it can make your bones become thin, weak, and very brittle. To strengthen the bones after treatment for hyperthyroidism, it is recommended to take calcium supplements and vitamin D. To get an idea of how much vitamin D you should be taking post-surgery, you can talk to your doctor for a recommendation.

Moving on from treatment, it is not unusual for a doctor to recommend their patients to an endocrinologist, who will be more specialized in the treatment of systems dealing with bodily hormones. You'll want to avoid stress at this stage as it can cause thyroid storm, which happens when a large amount of thyroid hormone gets released, resulting in a horrible and sudden worsening of any prior symptoms. Proper treatment is both recommended and effective at the prevention of thyroid storm, as well as other complications such as thyrotoxicosis.

In the long-term, the outlook for something like hyperthyroidism is dependent heavily on what is causing it. Some of the causes of hyperthyroidism can go away without ever seeking treatment. Whereas a more serious cause like Graves' disease is not to be taken lightly, as it will get much worse if it goes without treatment, and the complications due to Graves' disease are often life-threatening and will have an affect on your quality of life long-term. These are easy enough to subdue with proper care and an early diagnosis and treatment.

Hypothyroidism

Though we went over a little about hypothyroidism in chapter 1, it is important to take a closer look at the disorder, to gain a better idea of its symptoms, and proper treatment and care for it.

When the body is not producing enough of the thyroid hormones that it needs, this is what is known as hypothyroidism having occurred. This will cause the general functions of your body to become slowed down, as the thyroid gland is responsible for producing and secreting hormones which will provide energy to nearly every other portion of your body. Though this affliction can come to task at any age, it is more common for an underactive thyroid gland to be noticed in adults over the age of 60, as well as being more prevalent in women. A diagnosis of hypothyroidism is nothing to get too worked up about, fortunately, as treatment of hypothyroidism has been known to be quite effective, as well as being very simple and very safe.

Though the symptoms of having an underactive thyroid gland can vary from person to person, there is enough overlap in the symptoms for us to help lay out what to look out for. It is important to note, however, that there can be difficulty in pin-pointing that a symptom is that of hypothyroidism and that the severity of the condition itself plays a large role in which signs or symptoms will appear, as well as when they may make an appearance.

It is not at all uncommon for most people to experience the symptoms of this condition arriving in a slow progression over many years. The thyroid gland will grow ever slower and slower, which will only then allow the symptoms to be better identifiable. The trouble can become that many of the symptoms come with general aging, so if you suspect there is more to the picture, and that hypothyroidism is at play, it is important to go see a doctor. An example of some early symptoms which also come naturally with age are the symptomatic fatigue and gaining of weight.

If hypothyroidism does occur, however, other symptoms to keep an eye out for will be an uptick in depression, constipation, or muscle weakness. It is also common to begin becoming more sensitive to the cold, for the skin to become dry, and a reduction in sweating. Your heart rate will generally become slower, blood cholesterol may elevate, and joints may become stiff or experience more pain. It is also possible for memory to start becoming impaired, hair may thin or become dry. Your voice may become hoarse, muscles will stiffen and experience soreness, your face will become puffy and sensitive. In women, hypothyroidism as been known to negatively affect menstrual changes and cause difficulty in fertility.

When it comes to the causes of hypothyroidism, an autoimmune disease is fairly common to be the culprit at work. The body is designed in such a way that your immune system generally will protect the body's cells against any invading bacteria and virus. Therefore, when an unknown virus or bacteria enters the body, it is the immune system which will respond by sending out what are known as fighter cells, to destroy the foreign invading virus or bacteria.

However, it is not impossible for your body to begin confusing what are the healthy and normal cells, with the invading cells. This is what is then called an autoimmune response to the cells. And if this autoimmune response does not get properly treated, or if it is not properly regulated, it is your own immune system which will start to attack your healthy body tissues. Medically, this has been known to cause quite serious issues, which include hypothyroidism.

Hashimoto's disease, which we have mentioned before, is one such autoimmune condition that can occur, and it is the most common among the causes of having an underactive thyroid gland. The disease literally will attack the thyroid gland which will cause chronic thyroid inflammation, which, in turn, will reduce the functionality of the thyroid gland. As with Graves' disorder having links between generations, it is not at all uncommon to find that multiple members of a family have this same condition as well.

Hypothyroidism can even become an occurrence as a result of treatment for hyperthyroidism, which has the aim of lowering your thyroid hormone. It is not uncommon for the treatment to result in keeping the thyroid hormone too low, which then becomes hypothyroidism, which has been a known result of the radioactive iodine treatment for hyperthyroidism.

The surgical removal of the thyroid gland is yet another known cause of the occurrence of hypothyroidism. The entirety of the thyroid gland will be removed in the case of thyroid problems cropping up, which will affect the body's ability to produce thyroid hormone, and cause hypothyroidism. In this instance, you will typically be recommended to take thyroid medication for the rest of your life. In the case that it is only a smaller portion of the thyroid gland which is removed, it is possible for the thyroid gland to still be able to produce and secrete a healthy amount of hormones. In which case it will take a test of the blood to determine how much medication you will need.

It is possible for radiation therapy to be the cause if you have come down with hypothyroidism. A diagnosis of leukemia, neck cancer, or lymphoma will likely mean you have had to undergo a form of radiation therapy, which very nearly almost leads to the occurrence of hypothyroidism.

Just as possible, is a medication you may be taking to lower thyroid gland hormone production, to be the cause of hypothyroidism. Medications such as these are commonly used in the treatment of certain psychological diseases, and even have been known to be used in treating heart disease and cancer.

When it comes down the diagnosing of hypothyroidism, there are two primary methods which have been favored and work to best identify when it has occurred. The first being a strict medical evaluation, much like in the case of checking for hyperthyroidism. The doctor will give you a very thorough exam physically, as well as making sure to go over your medical history. Hypothyroidism has a couple physical signs which the doctor will be checking for primarily such as the dryness of the skin, how slow or quick your reflexes are, any swelling of the neck, and the rate of your heart beat. It is at this time that a doctor will also likely ask you to report any of the other symptoms listed earlier that you may have experienced, such as the depression, any fatigue, if you have been constipated, and a sensation of being more sensitive to the cold. It is also at this point it will be most helpful for you to let the doctor know of any thyroid conditions which have existed in your family.

To reliably get an idea of the existence of hypothyroidism in the body, it is required to conduct blood tests. It is only by this method that anyone will be able to tell and get a look at a measure of your body's thyroid-stimulating hormone levels, done by utilizing a thyroid-stimulating hormone test to see how much of the thyroid-stimulating hormone your pituitary gland is or is not creating. In the case that your thyroid gland is not producing enough of the hormone, the pituitary gland will respond to this by boosting the thyroid-stimulating hormone it produces in order to increase thyroid hormone production. If it turns out you have hypothyroidism, the levels of thyroid-stimulating hormone in your body will be increased, because your body is responding by making an attempt at stimulating more thyroid gland hormone activity. If hyperthyroidism is what ails you, the levels of the thyroid-stimulating hormone in your body will as having decreased, because in this case, your body has begun the process of attempting to halt the function of excessive production of the thyroid glands hormones.

Another useful method in the detection and diagnosis of hypothyroidism is to test the levels of T4 in the body, being produced by your thyroid gland, as T4 is produced directly by the thyroid gland. When they are used in conjunction with one another, a test of T4 levels and the thyroid-stimulating hormone test are very helpful in coming up with an evaluation of thyroid gland functionality. In general, if you the levels of thyroid-stimulating hormone in your body has increased, while the level of the hormone T4 has decreased, you much more than likely have hypothyroidism. Though, due to the sheer amount of conditions that can have such a negative impact on the thyroid gland, it could very well end up being necessary to conduct even more tests of the thyroid glands function I order to properly diagnose the issue.

Though it is true that for many people who have thyroid conditions, that the right amount of the proper medication will assist in the alleviation of their symptoms, you will have hypothyroidism for the rest of your life if you get it.

To get the best of hypothyroidism it is most commonly treated the best with the use of levothyroxine, also known as Levothroid or Levoxyl, which is T4 put into a synthetic form that is responsible for copying the action the thyroid hormone would regularly take if it were being produced as normal by your body. The idea behind doing this is that the medication will cause a return to the proper levels of the thyroid hormone in your blood. Once a restoration of the thyroid hormone level has occurred, many of the symptoms that come along with having hypothyroidism, will at the very least become much easier to manage, and at best the hypothyroidism symptoms will disappear altogether. It is important to expect it to take several weeks, following treatment, before relief sets in, and you start to feel a return to normalcy. There will also very likely be follow up appointments for testing your blood, which the doctor will recommend in order to keep a solid eye on your progress into recovery. Chances are that you will also receive some medication or other recommended methods to aid you in your recovery, be sure to speak with your doctor about the dosage you should be taking and to come up with a solid plan, that will most benefit you, for recovering in a timely fashion.

It is the case that many people who end up with hypothyroidism medicate for it, for the rest of their lives. Despite this, the dosage you will be taking thru ought that time is likely to go through changes. To better get an idea of how these dosages should be changing over time, it is best to get a check up on your thyroid-stimulation hormone levels every year. In this way, your doctor will be able to more properly adjust the amount you should be taking, or not taking, based on the blood levels indicated by the thyroid-stimulating hormone tests. Only by doing this regularly, will you and your doctor be able to achieve the recovery program that works best for you.

Plans and programs for this achievement may include medications and other hormone supplementation. Once again, synthetic versions of the hormone you need may be used, as they are a widely used and viable practice to aid in the recovery of hypothyroidism. The synthetic version of the hormone T3 is liothyronine, and T4 in its synthetic medication form is called levothyroxine, both of which act as suitable substitutes for their corresponding hormone.

If it was a deficiency in your iodine intake which caused your specific occurrence of hypothyroidism, it is likely that your doctor will recommend a supplementary form of iodine. Keep in mind to ask your doctor, and get the proper testing before taking anything, but selenium and magnesium supplements have been known to aid heavily in the treatment of hypothyroidism.

The golden ticket to any recovery or treatment is usually diet, and in the case of hypothyroidism, there is no exception. Though this is the case, and diet can be incredibly beneficial in your recovery and treatment, do not expect a change in your diet, doctor recommended or otherwise, to replace the need for a prescribed medication. Foods that are rich in selenium or magnesium such as nuts and seeds like the Brazil nut and sunflower seeds have been shown to be very beneficial additions to any diet to aid in the treatment of hypothyroidism.

Balance in your diet will play an especially important role, as the thyroid gland requires particular amounts of iodine in order to properly reach full functionality. There are foods such as whole grains, vegetables, fruits, and lean meats which can handily accomplish this without the need for iodine supplementation.

And of course, diet is only the beginning, exercise as well comes in as an important slice of the treatment and recovery pie. The muscle and joint pain that coincides with hypothyroidism will more often than not leave one to feel extreme fatigue and depression, both of which can be helped by creating and sticking to a regular work out regime. Though no exercise should be discounted, unless specifically told to avoid certain activities by your doctor, there are certain ones which will prove more beneficial than others for treating the symptoms of hypothyroidism. Low impact workouts such as swimming, riding a bike, doing Pilates or yoga, or even a good brisk walk, have been known to be very helpful low impact work outs that are helpful and easy to work in to a daily routine.

The building up of muscle mass by strength training, lifting weights, sit ups, pushups, and pull-ups, help reduce the lethargic feeling of sluggishness that comes along with hypothyroidism. The increase in muscle mass will result in an increase in the rate of your metabolism, which will simultaneously assist in decreasing any weight gain that the hypothyroidism may have caused.

And finally doing training that is primarily cardiovascular. As stated earlier, hypothyroidism is one of the ailments that can correlate with a heightened risk of having a cardiac arrythmia, or irregularity of the heartbeat. By taking steps to be more mindful of your cardiovascular health, exercising on a regular basis or schedule, will help in protecting your heart.

There are also alternative treatments which exist to help in taking care of hypothyroidism, such as animal extracts that contain the thyroid hormone. These extracts are made available from pigs because they contain both the thyroid hormone T4 and thyroid hormone T3. It is uncommon for these to be recommended, however, as they have not shown to be reliable in how to dose, as well as not being more effective than the typically recommended medications. It is also popular to find some glandular extracts in stores that are health food based. The risk that comes along with them is that the U.S. Food and Drug Administration plays no role in the monitoring or the regulation of these extracts. This has historically brought the guarantee of their pureness, legitimacy, and even their potency into question. If you decide to use these products, you do so at your own risk, but still be sure to inform your doctor so that they can adjust accordingly to your treatment.

You can go above and beyond in regards to hypothyroidism treatment, yet still deal with issues or complications that are longer lasting because of this harsh fluctuation to your body. Luckily there have been methods developed and used which will help to lessen the burden of hypothyroidisms effects on your life moving forward.

In the beginning, fatigue can feel like a lot to deal with, especially when associated with depression. These feelings can creep through even if you are taking proper dosages of your medication. It is of utmost importance that you get a good quality sleep every night to ease your treatment and recovery. A good, healthy diet, as well as the relief of stress through activities such as meditation, Pilates, and yoga, are effective strategies when it comes to combating lower energy levels.

It is also vitally important to recognize the difficulty of having a medical condition that is chronic, especially in the case of something like hypothyroidism, which comes along with its own mixed bag of other concerns to your overall health. Being able to talk about, or express, the experience of going through this will help. There are resources out there for support groups of other people who live with the effects of hypothyroidism, you can find a therapist to talk to, perhaps a close friend or loved one. Anyone who will be able to enable you to discuss your experience with openness and with honesty. You may even be able to receive a recommendation for meetings of people with hypothyroidism, from an education office at your local hospital. Connecting and communicating with others who can empathize with what you are going through could end up being an enormous aid in your recovery and life with hypothyroidism.

Important as well is making sure you monitor yourself for other health conditions that could arise. As we went over earlier, the main cause for hypothyroidism is an autoimmune disease. Just as well, links with hypothyroidism have also been found in conditions such as diabetes, having pituitary issues, having your sleep obstructed by sleep apnea, and lupus.

Just as with fatigue, depression is a common symptom and side effect of going through and living with hypothyroidism and should be watched closely. The thyroid glands hormone levels lower, the function of your body begins to slow down, and before you may realize it you are living with a depression that was not there before. It is vital to know what to look out for, and not just what, but also how to look after yourself while dealing with this.

Depression as a symptom can make hypothyroidism difficult to diagnose as there are many who may only experience difficulties or changes in mood as a symptom. It is for this reason, that instead of having a doctor check only your brain when checking for depression, it can also be important to ask them to check for signs of you having an underactive thyroid. Aside from the changes in mood, there are a few other similarities that exist in both having depression as well as hypothyroidism such as, gaining weight, finding it difficult to maintain concentration, feelings of daily fatigue, which coincide with a reduced desire and satisfaction with daily life, and hypothyroidism or depression could both effect your ability to sleep well.

Not all of their symptoms overlap so nicely though, both have their conditions which differentiate one from the other. In the case of hypothyroidism there are, of course, some physical signs such as the dryness of the skin, or the thinning and loss of hair. There is also the tendency to become constipated and the increase in levels of cholesterol.

These symptoms would be atypical if depression alone was the issue.

If you have hypothyroidism and it is the cause of your depression, then the correct treatment and care of the hypothyroidism should be just the remedy needed in order to treat your depression as well. If the hypothyroidism passes and depression remains, it may be important to talk to your doctor about receiving further help and a change in medication.

Along with depression being a symptom of hypothyroidism, it has recently been found, through studies, that around 60 percent or so of people who get hypothyroidism tend to also exhibit having anxiety as well. Studies are ongoing and are still growing in scope and size, though it would still be in your best interest to discuss all possibilities and symptoms with your doctor in order to more thoroughly and best tackle the treatment of hypothyroidism.

It cannot be stressed enough, how much of your body is under the affects and influence of your thyroid gland working properly to produce and secrete the correct levels of hormones. For this reason, when a woman gets hypothyroidism and simultaneously desires to get pregnant, she will be faced with her own subset of challenges to come. Have a low thyroid gland function during a pregnancy can cause a number of conflicts including various birth defects, have a still-birth or miscarriage, as well as anemia or a low birth weight. It is not uncommon for a woman with thyroid problems to have a perfectly healthy pregnancy, but to make sure that you reach this outcome it is important to do things such as eating well, keeping yourself informed about current and effective medicines, as well as talking to your doctor about testing.

Though testing may result in changes to your dosage or medication, it is also for this reason that it is important to make sure you are not deviating from the medications provided and the dosage your doctor has recommended.

Considering the thyroid issues adds on even more importance to the need for eating healthy while pregnant. Make sure that you are getting the proper amount of vitamins, minerals, and nutrients and consider taking multivitamins as well to supplement this.

It is not impossible to develop a thyroid issue such as hypothyroidism while pregnant. In fact, for every 1,000 pregnancies, this tends to occur in every 3 out of 5 women. It is important for doctors to routinely check thyroid levels during your pregnancy, as some will do, to make sure your thyroid levels aren't becoming to high or low. If they end up being higher or lower than they ought to be, it is likely that your doctor will recommend you starting treatment. Even some women who have never before had any thyroid issues may develop them once the baby is born, which is known as postpartum thyroiditis, and also tends to resolve itself after a year in around 80 percent of the women it shows up in. It is only the other 20 percent of women who will have this happen and then go on to require the long term treatment.

When hypothyroidism takes place, and the functions of the body slow down, it is quite typical for people to become prone to gaining weight, which is very likely due to what happens to the bodies ability to burn energy, which is that the efficiency to do so slows down as well. This change in the body will typically cause someone who has hypothyroidism to gain anywhere from 5 to 10 pounds in general, making the weight that is gained not entirely drastic, but someone could still find it quite alarming. It is very possible then, that once the hypothyroidism has been treated, that any weight gained will then be easily lost. If this does not occur, a simple change in diet, and adding regular exercise to your routine should aid in handily losing the weight, as your ability to manage weight will go back to normalcy, with the return to proper levels in your thyroid hormones.

Hypothyroidism is a common occurrence; therefore it is also commonly treated without issue. Hypothyroidism has been found to occur in around 4.6 percent of the American population that are 12 and older. Which comes out to about 10 million or so people who go on to live long healthy lives with the condition, and you may never even realize it. It is far more prevalent in people who are over the age of 60, and in women about 1 in 5 of them are likely to experience hypothyroidism by the time they have reached 60 years of age. One of the causes is Hashimoto's disease which happens to appear more in women who have reached middle-age, though it can absolutely show up in children and men. As Hashimoto's disease is hereditary, it is likely that if you get it, you did so from a relative, and have an increased chance then of passing it on down to your children.

It is important to keep an eye on your body, your health, and your thyroid gland as you get older. If, as the years go by, you begin to notice any of the changes gone over in this chapter so far, it is vital that you see a doctor in an attempt to get a proper diagnosis and seek treatment as soon as possible.

Hashimoto's Disease

Hashimoto's disease is an autoimmune disease which can be very destructive to your thyroid gland, and thereby your thyroid glands ability to function properly. Hashimoto's disease is also known as chronic autoimmune lymphocytic thyroiditis and is the most common cause of having an underactive thyroid gland, hypothyroidism, in the United States.

As an autoimmune disorder, Hashimoto's disease is one of many conditions that will be the cause of your body's white blood cells and your body's antibodies becoming confused and starting to attack the cells that make up the thyroid gland. What makes this happen precisely is still somewhat of a mystery to doctors, even still it is believed by some that factors of genetics may be involved.

With the cause of Hashimoto's disease being unknown, it is difficult to precisely put a finger on what puts a person at risk for having or contracting the disease. There are still, however, just a few factors that doctors are aware of which could signify being at risk for the disease. In the case of Hashimoto's disease, in particular, women happen to be seven times more likely to contract than men, and especially for women who have been pregnant before. Having a history of autoimmune diseases in the family is another factor that could mean you are at higher risk of having Hashimoto's at some point in your life, especially if the autoimmune diseases include Graves' disease, lupus, rheumatoid arthritis, if there is a history of Sjogren's syndrome in your family, or a history of type 1 diabetes, Addison's disease, and vitiligo. If it is the case that these autoimmune diseases are present in your family line or may have been based on symptoms of Hashimoto's disease, get together and discuss the possibility with your doctor, then make sure to get tested for the disease.

Hashimoto's disease is interesting in that the symptoms of it, are not symptomatic of Hashimoto's disease alone, in fact, they are similar to having the symptoms of an underactive thyroid gland, or hypothyroidism. Some signs to watch out for that your thyroid gland is not working properly to produce proper thyroid hormones, and that you may have Hashimoto's disease are your skin becoming dry and pale, constipation, if your voice becomes hoarse, you become depressed and start to feel sluggish or fatigued. High levels of cholesterol, a thinning of the hair, muscle weakness in the lower body, and intolerance to the cold may also be signs of hypothyroidism as a result of Hashimoto's disease. In women, it can also cause issues with fertility. Hashimoto's can exist inside of your body for many years before you begin to show any signs or symptoms, and during that time, it may progress while showing no signs of damage to the thyroid gland. Some with Hashimoto's disease end up with a goiter, an enlarging of the thyroid gland which causes the front of the neck to swell. Though generally painless, it is common for a goiter to make the act of swallowing difficult and for it to simulate a feeling of fullness in the throat.

Owing to it's difficulty to diagnose, your doctor may not suspect Hashimoto's of being prevalent until observing symptoms having hypothyroidism. In which case they will need to conduct a blood test designed to check the thyroid-stimulating hormone, or TSH, levels in your body. It is a relatively common and safe test, which is also an accurate way to check to see if you have Hashimoto's disease. Levels of thyroid-stimulating hormone are higher when the activity of the thyroid glad is lower because your body starts working harder to stimulate the production of more thyroid hormones to secrete from the thyroid gland. There are also blood tests that your doctor may conduct if they feel the need to check further for the levels of antibodies, cholesterol, and other thyroid hormones, T3 and T4, in your blood. Testing for all of these can help immensely in pinning down a diagnosis of Hashimoto's disease.

Unless your thyroid gland is functioning normally, in which case your doctor may still recommend regular checkups to monitor you for any changes, it is very likely that the need for treatment of Hashimoto's disease will be required.

The improper production of enough hormones in your body by your thyroid gland will likely result in the need to take medication. In the case of having to take this medication, it is also likely that you will be prescribed on it, though dose will vary, for the rest of your life. The effective drug most commonly prescribed is levothyroxine which is the hormone thyroxine, or T4, made synthetically, and which will successfully replace the missing hormone in your blood. The synthetic hormone drug levothyroxine tends not to have any noticeable side effects, and regular use has been known to frequently return the hormone levels of the body back to normal, restoring proper function of the thyroid gland. When this happens, all other symptoms of Hashimoto's disease and hypothyroidism generally tend to disappear altogether, though it is likely that your doctor will still recommend that you still get regular testing done so that your hormone levels can be consistently monitored to prevent something like hypothyroidism from becoming a problem again moving forward. Getting the regular testing allows the doctor to adjust the dosage of your medication as necessary if at all necessary.

It is important to consider before going on levothyroxine, that there are supplements and medications which will have an effect on your body's ability to absorb the drug. As such, make sure you have a discussion about this with your doctor if you are taking any other medications, especially if they include iron or calcium supplements, or estrogen. Some medications for cholesterol have been known to cause an issue, as well as proton pump inhibitors which are used as a treatment for acid reflux.

Though these have been known to cause an issue, there is what could be an easy work around of simply changing what time of the day you take your other medicines in conjunction with the doctor recommended thyroid medicine. It is also possible that certain foods could end up being involved in the efficacy of your thyroid medicine. It is best to discuss all of this with your doctor to come up with an efficient way for you to take your thyroid medicine, based on your dietary needs.

The severity of complications due to leaving Hashimoto's untreated varies and are not worth the risk if you ever contract, or if you have it. They go far beyond just hypothyroidism and include heart problems that an include total failure of the heart. It is not unusual for anemia to be a result of leaving Hashimoto's disease unattended. Depression and a decrease in libido are common, as well as higher levels of cholesterol in the blood and experiencing a sense of confusion or loss of consciousness.

Hashimoto's disease has also been the culprit responsible for complications during a woman's pregnancy cycle. It is far more likely, that if you carry out a pregnancy while having untreated Hashimoto's disease, that you may be putting your child at higher risk of being born with defects of their kidneys, their heart, and even their brains.

These complications can be limited by talking to your doctor during the pregnancy and keeping on top of monitoring your thyroid glands hormone levels with the proper blood testing. If you are a pregnant woman and have thyroid issues, such preventative measures could mean a severe change in the life and health of your child. However, if you have not had any known disorders with your thyroid or hormone levels, it is not recommended that you get regular or constant screening done during the pregnancy.

Graves' Disease

Another autoimmune disorder, Graves' disease is responsible for causing your thyroid gland too create too much of the thyroid hormones in your body. When this happens it is a condition referred to commonly as hyperthyroidism. Graves' disease, is named such for the man who discovered it, an Irish physician named Robert J. Graves, and is regarded as one of the most common forms hyperthyroidism takes, having an effect on around 1 out of every 200 people.

When Graves' disease occurs in the body, it will cause your immune system to begin creating antibodies that are known as thyroid-stimulating immunoglobulins, that attach themselves to the body's usually healthy cells of the thyroid gland. By doing this they end up causing the thyroid gland to produce and secrete more of the thyroid hormones than it is meant to for your body. The hormones that are produced by the thyroid gland go on to affect a great number of your body's functions including its temperature, the function of the nervous system, the development of the brain, and the list goes on. For this reason, hyperthyroidism can end up having a negatively driven affect on not just all of those functions, but when left untreated can also cause the loss of weight and mental and physical fatigue. Hyperthyroidism has also been found to be responsible for such things as depression and emotional liability where the individual will uncontrollably cry or laugh or put on other manic emotional displays.

Due to the role that Graves' disease can invariably play on the appearance of hyperthyroidism in the body, it is no surprise that the two would contain a sharing of many of the same symptoms. These symptoms include tremors especially of the hands, a loss of weight, tachycardia, which is the rapidity in the rate of the heart, becoming intolerant to heat or warmth, fatigue, nervousness and irritability, the swelling of the front of the neck, due to the enlargement of the thyroid gland, known as a goiter, an increase in the frequency of having bowel movements, as well as diarrhea, weakness of the muscles, and having it become difficult to get a good full night's worth of sleep. Among the people who experience having Graves' disease, it is only a small percentage who will experience the skin thickening around their shin area and become reddened, an affliction which is known as Graves' dermopathy.

Another common symptom of Graves' disease which one may go through while experiencing the condition, is what is called Graves' ophthalmopathy. Graves' ophthalmopathy is what occurs when the eyes of the afflicted individual appear to be enlarged, which is a result of the eyelids retracting. When Graves' ophthalmopathy happens, it is entirely possible that your eyes may begin to bulge outwards from your eye sockets. Estimates say that as much as 30 percent of the people who end up developing Graves' disease will observe at least a mild case of what is known as Graves' ophthalmopathy and that for up to 5 percent of the people will instead experience an extreme case of the eye bulging.

Because of autoimmune diseases such as Graves' disease, the immune system will begin to fight against what are the healthy cells and healthy tissues of the body. Normally, your immune system is producing proteins which are known as antibodies, which are responsible for fighting against foreign invaders to your body, the likes of harmful viruses and bacteria. The antibodies produced this way are formed especially with the duty of targeting a specific invader to the host. When it comes to the effect of Graves' disease on the body, your immune system begins to mistake healthy thyroid cells as these foreign harmful cells and produces the thyroid-stimulating immunoglobulins which then mistakenly go off to attack what are your healthy thyroid cells.

Scientists and doctors alike, are aware that it is indeed possible for a person to have inherited the ability for their body to make antibodies which then go against their own healthy cells, yet they have made no determination that such an occurrence is what is the cause for Graves' disease, or who will end up developing Graves' disease.

Despite that though, there are experts who believe that they have been able to button down on some factors which may increase ones risk for the development of graves disease which includes its tendency to be hereditary. So be sure to discuss family medical history with your doctor and talk about whether or not there are family members who have, or who ay have had Graves' disease. It is also believed by these experts that stress, gender, and someone's age may be some of the facets that end up putting someone at higher risk of getting Graves' disease. It is typical for the disease to be found in people who are younger than the age of 40, and it has been more prevalent, about seven to eight times so, in women rather than men.

Having had, or having still, another autoimmune disease is yet another factor that will increase your risk of ever getting Graves' disease. Examples of such autoimmune diseases are having Crohn's disease, rheumatoid arthritis, and diabetes mellitus, among others.

For the diagnosing of Graves' disease, when it is suspected, it is not unheard of for your doctor to request lab tests. The use of your families medical history as well, especially if there is a case of someone in your family having had Graves' disease, will be able to help act as a basis for your doctor to zero in on diagnosing whether you have Graves' disease as well or not. This is something that thyroid gland blood tests will be needed for in order to confirm. Your doctor may request that these tests and others may be handled by a specialist expert in diseases which are related to the body's hormones, known as an endocrinologist, in order to help get the diagnosis of Graves' disease. Other tests which your doctor may request are full bloodwork tests, a thyroid gland scan, an uptake test utilizing radioactive iodine, a test for levels of TSH, or thyroid stimulating hormone, and a TSI test, which is the thyroid-stimulating immunoglobulins.

By combining the efforts of the endocrinologist, as well as the array of tests, it is more possible for your doctor to determine if you do indeed have and need treatment for Graves' disease specifically, or if another thyroid disorder is what is at work, and thus requires its own specific form of treatment.

There are a number of options available for treatment when someone is diagnosed as having Graves' disease. These are generally the taking of anti-thyroid drugs, therapy in the form of RAI, or radioactive iodine, and getting thyroid gland surgery. It is not abnormal for a doctor, in the case of Graves' disease, to recommend, all, two, or just one of the treatments for the afflicted.

When it comes to treatment via anti-thyroid drugs, you will typically be taking medications such as methimazole, which is taken orally as a tablet and works by putting a stop to the thyroid gland producing and secreting too much thyroid hormone, and propylthiouracil, which is also taken orally and generally used as a back up if a drug like methimazole did not end up working well enough. The use of beta-blockers is also recommended on occasion as they are used in assistance of reducing the effects of symptoms until another treatment method can start working.It is radioactive iodine treatment, or RAI, which is among the most common treatments suggested to those suffering of Graves' disease. It is required, during this treatment, that the individual seeking treatment take specified doses of radioactive iodine-131, the purpose of which is to destroy thyroid cells. The radioactive iodine-131 will be ingested orally, in small amounts, via pill. Be sure to discuss with your doctor and risks or precautions that come with this treatment.

The less frequent option for treatment is the thyroid surgery. This treatment will tend to be a last resort if the other options have not worked to full capacity, if there is a reason to be suspect of thyroid cancer being present, or if the patient is a pregnant woman who is unable to take any of the regularly prescribed anti-thyroid drugs.

In the case of surgery being necessary, it is not uncommon the doctor to issue the removal of your thyroid gland completely, in the interest of preventing the return of the hyperthyroidism. In which case, thyroid hormone replacement surgery will be necessary on a regular basis. Talk to your doctor about the possible side effects of choosing to go through with surgery, as well as generally what to expect moving forward

Goiter

A goiter, goitre, thyroid cyst, or Plummer's disease, is a general term used for when there is an observable enlargement of the thyroid gland, usually resulting in a noticeable swelling of the front of the neck. Treatment for a goiter can be handled in a variety of ways, and the treatment method is dependent on the goiters location, the length of its presence, and how exactly it is affecting the thyroid glands performance.

Though usually unable to be seen or even felt, the thyroid gland generally tends to become detectable by touch and even perceptible to the eye when there is a goiter present. An expanse of the thyroid gland, or goiter, can be the cause of the whole thyroid gland expanding, which is known as a "smooth goiter", or just a part of the thyroid gland expanding, which is also called a "cystic" or "nodular" goiter. A goiter is not a sure symptom of having an active thyroid, known as hyperthyroidism, or underactive thyroid, known as hypothyroidism, and, in fact, the majority of people who have a goiter, retain a perfectly normal use of their thyroid gland.

A number of reasons exist for the existence of a goiter. Among these are included a deficiency in your levels of iodine. Iodine may be a trace element, but it is far from trivial. It assists in helping the thyroid gland in maintaining proper functionality and making the thyroid glands hormones. There are two primary hormones which are produced and secreted by the thyroid gland, these are T4 or thyroxine, and T3, also known as triiodothyronine. The approximate number of people who have iodine deficiency comes out to about 2.2 billion and it is estimated that around 29 percent of the worlds total population live in an area that is considered to be deficient in iodine. It is reported that people in the U.K. have proper levels of iodine as a part of their regular diet. If you are keeping your eye out for food sources that are a good source of iodine, there are salts that have iodine supplements, as well, non-organic milk is plentiful with iodine.

Thyroiditis is anther well known cause of goiter. Thyroiditis is more commonly referred to as when the thyroid gland has become inflamed. Around the world, the most common reason for thyroiditis occurring is Hashimoto's disease, or Hashimoto's thyroiditis, which is an autoimmune disease that causes the bodies antibodies to start to become confused and begin attacking healthy cells of the thyroid gland. Hashimoto's disease is not the only cause of the thyroiditis condition though, it could also stem from viral infection, and has been known to occur just after or during pregnancy.

A goiter has also been known to occur due to Graves' disease, another autoimmune disease, this one causing the immune systems antibodies attacks on thyroid cells to make the thyroid gland overactive, resulting in hyperthyroidism. It is this hyperthyroidism, or over activity of the thyroid glands capacity for producing and secreting hormones, which is the cause of the swelling of the thyroid gland.

If there are benign growths on the thyroid gland, they have been known to cause a goiter, most commonly known for doing this is a follicular adenoma, which can be a firm or rubbery tumor surrounded by a fibrous capsule.

External factors that may be the cause of goiter are known as goitrogens. Included among what would be considered a goitrogen are medicines such as the mental health drug lithium, and cabbage type vegetables. Ingestion in the excess of these vegetables, which include cassava or kelp, will likely result in the growth formation of a goiter.

There are physiological demands put on the body during pregnancy and during puberty which have been known to be at the root of a goiter. And as with other causes like Graves' disease and Hashimoto's disease, there is a strong likelihood of inherited genetic reasons that one may at some point experience goiter.

Due to the varying reasons for the existence of goiter, there are also a multiplicity of types of goiter. The first of these types is known as colloid goiter, or endemic goiter, which is a development due directly to a lack of sufficient iodine levels. As a result, the people who tend to end up with a colloid goiter are those we mentioned, who live somewhere with a less dense supply of iodine.

The next type of goiter is the nontoxic goiter, or sporadic goiter, as it is also well known. Though the definite cause of a goiter of this type is regarded as generally unknown, it is surmised that a sporadic goiter is a result of taking medications, such as lithium, for example, or so it is believed. Among the may uses for lithium, it is perhaps most commonly recognized as the drug used for aiding in the treatment of mood based disorders, the likes of bipolar or depression. The nontoxic name is apt in regard to this form of goiter, as they are benign, and have no discernable effect on the production or secretion function of the thyroid gland, leaving the thyroid to function at a healthy and normal capacity.

The final type of commonly recognized goiter is known as the toxic nodular or multinodular goiter. Generally originating and taking form from as merely an extension from what was a simple goiter prior, the toxic nodular goiter will take the form of at least one, but often more, small nodules on the expanding thyroid gland. This toxic nodular goiter, having taken a sort of root on the thyroid gland, then begins to produce its own thyroid hormone, which plays a big part in the causation of hyperthyroidism.

As mentioned above, it can be difficult to detect goiter before it has really taken effect to the thyroid gland, but after it has begun doing it's work it is most common for it to cause a swelling of the front of the neck, making it clearly visible as well as felt. Before the expanding has commenced, it is common to have had nodules existing in your thyroid gland, these small nodules cannot be felt, and may have even been only a chance occurrence due to examinations, and of scans, that were applied for other reasons. Cases such as these are rather common, and when they occur, there has been a tendency to notice no sign of a goiter up to that point. As nodules appear on the thyroid, ranging from smaller nodules to much larger nodules, it is the presence of these nodules which is what is the cause of noticeable swelling of the neck.

This swelling and the nodules which are collecting on the thyroid gland cause other symptoms to occur, like having a difficult time of swallowing or of trying to breathe, it is not uncommon for coughing to be a symptom, your voice may start to become hoarse, and there may be a dizzy sensation that is noticeable when you raise an arm above your head.

Goiter is a rather common occurrence. It is calculated by the World Health Organization, that around the world, goiter affects nearly 12 percent of the global population. However, it has also been recorded that in Europe, the rate of goiter is lower by a slight amount. Goiter being considered endemic, or noticeably affecting a certain area is a common occurrence wherever iodine is scarce, and the endemic definitions are only applied when goiter is recognized on 1 out of 10 people within a certain population.

It is usual for goiter to be the diagnosis when there is noticeable swelling on the neck that can be seen without the need of a scan, also making it detectable with the touch of the hand, due to the enlarged thyroid gland in your neck, something a doctor will be quick to check for, likely before anything else.

There are also a number tests a general practitioner may order in order to examine the levels in your blood of thyroid hormones coming from the thyroid gland, as well as wanting to make sure of the levels of antibodies that are prevalent in the bloodstream. This examination will often take the form of blood tests, that are used to detect the changes in levels of the hormones as well as whether or not the level of production of the antibodies has increased, which tends to happen in response to the body experiencing an injury or infection in the blood.

A thyroid scan, or thyroid uptake scan, will show the size of the goiter itself, as well as what condition the goiter is in. It will also aid in identifying any differences in activity, in various places on the thyroid gland.

A biopsy may be recommended, the procedure of which involves removing samples of your thyroid gland, and then sending the samples of your thyroid gland's tissue to an outside laboratory or endocrinologist for examination.

It is also possible that an ultrasound scan may be used which will help for a doctor to see images of the inside of your neck, getting a much closer look at the size of the invasive goiter, allowing for the observation of nodules. As more ultrasounds are done, it is even then possible to track the changes in size or shape of the nodules, and the size of the goiter.

You may, at some point, be referred to an endocrinologist in order to get an outpatient assessment, giving you and the doctor more information from the examination by an expert. During their examination you may have to undergo a test known as a fine needle aspiration, which is done on the thyroid gland. For the procedure to take place, the endocrinologist will make use of a fine needle which, utilizing the guiding sight of an ultrasound, will be used to remove tissue from your thyroid gland, only a small amount will be needed. The tissue removed from your thyroid gland is then studied under the lens of a microscope, which will assist the endocrinologist in assessing exactly the types of cells which are currently present in your thyroid gland. It is not at all uncommon for a procedure like this to need to be repeated one or more times, for the sake of reaching an accurate result and helping you on your way to treatment and recovery.

There is no one, cut and dry, blanket method for treating a goiter, as the treatment will depend entirely on precisely what is the cause that is underlying the goiter. As well, a particular course of action will be decided by your doctor on the basis of the size of the goiter, and the condition that the goiter is in, as well as the symptoms you have that are associated with the goiter. It will also be important to not overlook any factors to your health that may have been responsible for the goiters formation when looking into treatment options.

A goiter which can be regarded as simple, having a prevalence of causing no imbalances in the thyroid gland, as well as no seeming problems as a result of the thyroid gland, will be less likely to cause further obstructions or overall issues.

In order to shrink a goiter, in the case of hypo or hyperthyroidism, it may be enough to just take prescribed medicines as a treatment for the symptoms and for the swelling of the thyroid gland. Medications which are known as corticosteroids often see use in the task of reducing any inflammation, or when there is a prevalence of thyroiditis.

Medicinal treatments for a goiter are not always the most effective response, however. It is not at all uncommon for a goiter to have grown too large to be able to respond properly to medicinal therapy and begin to shrink. In such a case there are surgeries which are available, known as a thyroidectomy. Undergoing a thyroidectomy will mean removing your thyroid gland completely and is a common option for when the thyroid gland grows too large and further obstructs what would otherwise be simple actions, such as swallowing or breathing.

When you are going through the experience of trying to treat what is the most harmful of the goiter family, the toxic nodular or multinodular goiter, RAI, or radioactive iodine treatment is typically the necessary response. You will be given a tablet, the RAI, which is a small amount of the radioactive iodine, which gets ingested orally and begins the process of destroying thyroid gland tissue.

When it comes to the treatment of a goiter, there are options for home care which can be very helpful and ought not to be overlooked as such. When you have finished up with all the treatment that can be offered at the hospital, or by a referred endocrinologist, it is an entirely common possibility that a discussion with your general practitioner will end in him or her suggesting you continue care of yourself in the home, with a prescription of some form of medication, which may end up being a decrease or increase in the amounts of iodine that you are ingesting regularly. This will, of course, be determined by the type of goiter that was ailing you, as well as requiring regular testing to keep an eye on your iodine levels, and the efficiency of your thyroid glands production and secretion of hormones. If it all ends up that a goiter is non-problematic, being too small to count as an issue or cause an imbalance, you may require no treatment or care at home at all.

Conclusion

So now you know all about Bariatric surgery. The different kinds of procedures and how they differ, how to prepare for it and what recovery will be like. If you are just starting out and trying to get information, I hope this helped you and once again congrats on taking the first step to a new and healthier life. If you are preparing for surgery, I hope this has helped you with your preparations and can make you feel more secure knowing what to expect on the day of your procedure. If you are currently in recovery, then this should have helped you with your diet and physical restrictions and what you are capable of doing right now. This book should also have given you an estimate of how much weight you can expect to lose from each type of procedure. Please keep in mind that any weight loss surgery can only help you to lose weight. You must be the one who wants to change and follow through with your plans. Surgery is not going to change your lifestyle, habits, addictions or any other cause of your obesity.

The next step is to choose some of the recipes that appeal to you and start cooking! If you have completed your bariatric surgery, please be sure that you follow all post-operative instructions from your doctor or surgeon. If you have yet to complete your surgery, then take this time to try out a few of the recipes in this book and choose your favorites. You can go grocery shopping and be stocked up on all of the ingredients you will need after your surgery. You might even decide to cook ahead of time and make some freezer meals that will be easy to reheat after your surgery is complete. After your weight loss surgery, you will be making a complete lifestyle change. To that end, all of the recipes are suitable for meal prepping and can benefit you in packing breakfasts, lunches, and snacks that you can take along with you if you go to work or school.

For this is not truly the end is it, but merely a small step in a forward direction. It is now time to utilize what you have learned going through these pages, and all that the knowledge contained within has to offer. If you or a loved one you know has, has had, or may seem to have a thyroid issue, every tool that is needed to aid them or yourself in the journey forward is now at your fingertips.

Now is when it is time to go see a doctor, to make sure that information is properly communicated. It is never too late, and never a bad idea, especially where the thyroid gland is concerned, to set oneself up with a regular and balanced diet, as well as having a plan for daily exercise in a range of activities.

Again, thank you so much for reading, I wish you all the best moving forward, and if you enjoyed the book, please leave a favorable review on amazon.